SIT-UPS
ARE STUPID
& CRUNCHES
ARE CRAP

SIT-UPS ARE STUPID
&CRUNCHES ARE CRAP

How to Strengthen Your
Core, Get Great Abs, and
Conquer Back Pain

DR. TODD SINETT

EAST END PRESS

SIT-UPS ARE STUPID AND CRUNCHES ARE CRAP:
How to Strengthen Your Core, Get Great Abs, and Conquer Back Pain

Copyright © 2020 by Todd Sinett

Published by
EAST END PRESS
Bridgehampton, NY

ISBN: 9781732491243
Ebook ISBN: 9781732491250

First Edition

Book Design by Neuwirth & Associates
Cover Design by Neuwirth & Associates

Manufactured in the United States of America

10 9 8 7 6 5 4 3 2 1

CONTENTS

PART ONE
THE THEORY WHY SIT-UPS ARE
STUPID AND CRUNCHES ARE CRAP

PART TWO
NO PAIN, BIG GAIN!

Larry Ellison, the founder of Oracle, once said, "When you innovate, you've got to be prepared for everyone telling you [that] you are nuts." Well, quite frankly, I am feeling nutty.

INTRODUCTION

TITLE GOT YOUR attention? Good—because you should never do a sit-up or any version of a crunch ever again. Don't do them with your legs up, don't do them with your legs down, don't do them on a ball, don't do them against a wall, simply don't ever do them at all!

Conventional wisdom says abdominal and core training should consist of sit-ups and crunches. Trainers, professional athletes, and the average exerciser follow this approach, but working your abs and core according to these training practices is downright harmful. The truth is that doing sit-ups and crunches is physiologically reckless.

But don't worry: there are other, healthier ways to get great abs, and this book will teach you the proper ways to get them without compromising your back and neck health.

. . .

First things first. Who am I, and how am I qualified to tell you how to work out your abs? What makes me more knowledgeable than your fitness trainer who has you drop and do 100 crunches? Here's my story:

My name is Dr. Todd Sinett, and I am a second-generation chiropractor, as well as a certified fitness trainer. I happened to have a father who was one of the most innovative doctors I have ever known. My father would say that he wasn't always this way but rather learned his inquisitive approach when, as a chiropractor, he suffered from severe debilitating back pain that kept him bedridden for nine months. Frustrated that every known profession was treating him unsuccessfully, including his own, he studied everything there is to know about back pain from bed.

Thankfully, he finally found a doctor with a different approach. This doctor found that sugar, which was a staple of my father's diet, irritated his digestive system and caused his severe back spasms. Turns out, anything that can upset the digestive system can reflex and then affect the muscular system of the back.

Though certainly skeptical, my father was willing to try anything. He completely changed his diet, and within two weeks my father was cured.

The doctor, aptly named Dr. Goodheart, reasoned that the majority of people lead unhealthy lifestyles. If you follow the vast majority, you will be resigned to live an unhealthy life, too, he said. He encouraged my father to see with his own eyes, listen with his own ears, and not be afraid to go against the grain. Well, my father spent his entire professional career doing just that, and in 1995 I joined my father in practice, armed with my very own inquisitive approach.

INTRODUCTION

In 2008, my father (before his passing) and I wrote a book called *The Truth About Back Pain*, which explains that the vast majority of us suffer from back pain because we only receive one-third of the diagnosis and treatment options. Our premise is that back pain comes from not one but three sources:

1. Structural issues such as muscles, discs, and bones
2. Nutritional issues (remember, we are what we eat)
3. Emotions or stress

If you only address one factor of back pain, it makes it impossible to successfully treat back pain.

As both my father's reputation and my own grew, patients would not just seek us out for their back problems but also for many other physical ailments, such as headaches, foot pain, neck pain, groin problems, and more. Professional athletes, famous movies stars, and business leaders were looking for our help for their myriad ailments. I have treated people on the sidelines of major sporting events, been flown to movie sets, and have worked backstage at Madison Square Garden before a sold-out show.

I am sharing with you my background not to impress you but rather to impress upon you that, as Dr. Goodheart said, the majority of people—even famous people—lead unhealthy lifestyles. Most people, I have seen, know little about properly training their abdominals. I have worked with professional athletes, dancers, and trainers, and regardless of their access to the "best training practices," they, too, are suffering from core imbalance. I am not some trainer who is writing an abs book just because they train a famous person—I am a doctor who is writing an abs book because I have seen way too many people who have great-looking abs and terrible back pain.

For the past twenty-five years, I have been working with a vast majority of patients ultimately suffering from imbalanced cores. I can no longer sit idly by and let destructive exercise practices (namely sit-ups and crunches) continue to dominate our workouts. What is vital to understand is that there are healthy ways to obtain great-looking abs and unhealthy ways to obtain them.

After the release of *The Truth About Back Pain*, I continued to fine-tune my theories and treatments for back pain and published a self-diagnostic and treatment book called *3 Weeks to a Better Back* in 2016 and *The Ultimate Backbridge Stretch Book*, a photo stretch book that allows you to safely and gently stretch any part of your body, in 2017. For a lot of people, flexibility is a missing link to health, and *The Ultimate Backbridge Stretch Book* helps you reclaim your posture, alignment, and flexibility. I also published a book in 2018 called *The Back Pain Relief Diet*, which elaborates on the undiscovered key of back pain: your diet.

I have explored the various causes of back pain in my books, but I decided I wanted to write an entire book dedicated to the abs and our current exercise regime. Why? Because core work is one of the leading structural causes of back and neck pain that most doctors never explore. Again, *why*? Because everyone assumes exercise is healthy and that fitness instructors know what they are talking about.

This book is intended to hone in deeper on the structure of your body, highlight core imbalance as caused by your current abdominal workout regimen, and give you different, healthier exercises for your body and your back. Every body is unique, but one thing I've realized is that almost nobody should be doing sit-ups or crunches.

My book will provide you with the road map on how to get great-looking abs in a way that maintains core balance. This book is for:

1. Anyone who wants to lose their gut, get healthy abs, a balanced core, and better posture, and heal their pain.

2. Anyone who is looking for a great workout guide for any fitness level, from the beginners all the way up to the fitness experts.

3. The couch potato and the person who never wanted to do sit-ups or crunch exercises in the first place. This book is your validation not to do them. While I do hope it will inspire you to get flat abs in a healthier way, I am pretty happy to help you stick it to that exercise know-it-all.

DIAGNOSIS: CORE IMBALANCE

BACK IN ABOUT 2003, I was examining a patient named Jenifer who was suffering from neck, upper back, and low back pain. She had been suffering for quite a while, and her pain only seemed to be getting worse and worse by the week. Chiropractors, physical therapists, massage therapists, and orthopedists had previously treated her, but her pain persisted at a 9 on a scale of 10 without any relief. She was tight and stiff all over, barely able to turn her head or bend to tie her shoes.

Jenifer wasn't your average out-of-shape person. In fact, she was the exact opposite: she was an ESPN fitness model who did workouts on the network's shows. When I examined her, I was surprised to see that her posture was out of alignment. I also noticed, when checking her muscular function, that her resistance was quite poor.

None of this made any sense because she was the picture of health and fitness—the example of what we all strive to look like. I asked myself how someone so healthy looking could be so unhealthy. How could someone who appeared to be so strong actually be so weak?

I asked her about her work on the fitness shows, and she said that at the end of every show, for at least 10 minutes, she would do hundreds of sit-ups and crunches. She did hundreds of these shows a year, so this added up to a lot of sit-ups.

Could it be that the sit-ups and crunches were making her sick? I had been studying the effects of extension therapy and wondered what would happen if I had her lie down over a big exercise ball to put her spine into extension. When I went and got one of those large exercise balls from my therapy room and had her stretch over it as if she were doing a bridge, she immediately exclaimed, "This feels great!" The extension provided her a stretch and relief that she hadn't had in months.

Upon reexamining her after lying over the ball, her pain dramatically decreased and flexibility dramatically improved. I diagnosed her problem as core imbalance brought on by too much forward posture caused by all the sit-ups and crunches. To discover that her *exercise was causing her core imbalance, resulting in pain* was mind-boggling to me.

I was so blown away by this discovery that I immediately got my father, who was practicing just down the hall from me. I had him lie over the exercise ball so that he could feel the effects—only to have him fall off!

Off to the drawing board I went: I created a product called Backbridge that was safe for anyone to use. Backbridge comes with five varying levels to allow the user to find the proper amount of stretch for their own spine. (You'll learn more about Backbridge in Section 9 of the book.)

Armed with this new discovery, I continued to examine patients and found that it wasn't just my athlete patients who suffered from core imbalance. It was just about everyone. Unfortunately, more than 90 percent of all people—from the out-of-shape administrative assistant to the professional athlete—are walking around with core imbalance, which creates significant postural issues and altered biomechanics.

Why do so many of us have an imbalanced core? Think about it: we spend our days hunched forward in front of computers, sitting in our cars commuting, watching television, bent down staring at our smartphones, and the list goes on and on. Crunches and sit-ups cause us to hunch forward even more. These are the last exercises we should want to do.

FAST FACTS ABOUT CORE IMBALANCE

1. Sit-ups and crunches create a shortening of our abdominals by causing too much forward pull, called flexion.
2. Forward pull (flexion) creates core and postural imbalance.
3. Core and postural imbalance lead to altered biomechanics, creating pain, weakness, and injuries.
4. Core imbalance greatly contributes to non-contact injuries.

Chances are that you are suffering from core imbalance, too. Take this test, and find out:

■

THE CORE IMBALANCE TEST

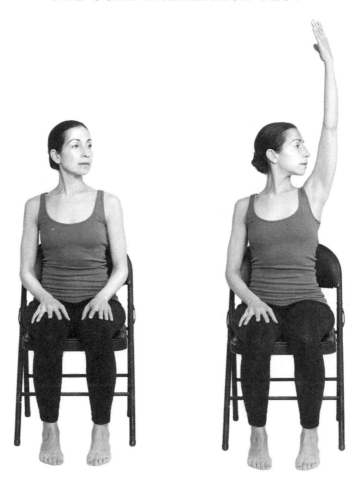

1. Turn your head to one side and see how far you can see.

2. Raise your arms above your head and turn your head to the same side again.
3. If you can see further with your arms above your head, you have core imbalance.

If you have core imbalance, raising your arms above your head allows you to stretch the abdominal muscles—exactly the opposite of flexion—which is why you can see further. In other words, if your body functions better with your arm above your head, it means that your core is restricting its function, resulting in imbalance and, subsequently, pain.

Your range of motion should be the same when you turn your head with your arms down or up in the air. If your range of motion is the same, but you still have neck pain, you may have a neck strain caused by sleeping funny, stress and tension, or clenching your teeth.

STRAIN VS. TRAIN

My studies while working with patients led me onto a new path of observation and revealed that sit-ups and crunches strain, rather than train, our abs. What a difference a letter makes!

As a doctor, it is my job to help people recover from their injuries, but I believe that it is even more important to help prevent them in the first place. *Doctor* in Latin means, "to teach," and I will teach you in this book how to properly train your core without introducing pain, weakness, and injury to your body. Terms such as *stretch, loosen, lengthen,* and *relax* are just as important as *strength* and will be key to safely and effectively training.

While doing my research for this book, I was both relieved to find that numerous well-esteemed colleagues share my view that our abdominal and core training is misguided at best, as well as a bit disappointed to find that my theories aren't completely original. The vast majority of "How To" articles I found in reference to getting great abs were focused on abdominal appearance and not the core's interrelationship to one's anatomy. This led me to numerous back pain and rehabilitation books to really study the anatomy of the abdominals.

I dove deeper into concepts such as anatomy trains, fascial lines, and anatomical connectedness: in layman's terms, how every muscle, tendon, and ligament is intertwined and related. An imbalance in one's feet or hips could create a cascade of imbalance leading to pain and significant injuries elsewhere in the body.

This led me to think about non-contact injuries and a question I would repeatedly ask myself when specifically treating athletes: How could a professional athlete who is supposed to be so fine-tuned suffer a debilitating injury from the most mundane task, like bending over just to pick up their sports ball? The answer for the vast majority of these cases was that these athletes were suffering from imbalanced cores—and that the repetitive movements with an imbalanced core compounded over time, resulting in tears and big problems.

I know what I have to say may be a bit controversial, but as you read you will realize it is simply common sense: sit-ups *are* stupid and crunches *are* crap. Exercise is supposed to release our body. Sit-ups and crunches create more flexion, which just makes the rectus abdominus shorter and shorter. This is especially true for people with larger bellies who add flexion on their abdominal muscles by pulling them forward with excess weight. To release the strain on your abs, you need to exercise with extension. This entire book is based on the science of flexion and the lack of extension our spines get in modern daily life, as well as the pain that's being caused as a result.

My research is largely based on the work of Dr. Stuart McGill of Waterloo University in books such as *Ultimate Back Fitness* and *Performance and Back Mechanics*. Over the past few decades, he has written extensively on the topic of back injuries and the concept of core stability. He describes the core as your home base: it involves not just the muscles of your abs but also your back muscles, your buttocks and hip muscles, and your chest muscles. No one can afford to neglect this building block of the body, and proper core training is the underpinning of fundamental human motion.

The rest of the book is broken into two parts. The first part is the theory behind *Sit-Ups Are Stupid and Crunches Are Crap*. You'll learn about how "The Business of Abs" has led you to spot-train your abs while completely disregarding the anatomy of the body, causing you to have back, neck, and shoulder pain. You'll learn how the ab muscles actually work and why your workout is failing you. And you'll learn to reverse your own core imbalance with gentle healing stretches and get tips for improving posture. Regaining your core balance will help your flexibility, breathing, and digestion and prevent non-contact injuries, as well as ease pain you are currently experiencing.

The second part provides you with a proper exercise routine and meal guide to help you get the abs you always wanted without hurting yourself. You'll learn why you need a four-pronged approach of cardiovascular training, strength training, core exercises, and healthy eating to get that flat, awesome-looking stomach. My No-Crunch Workout is core-friendly to help strengthen your back and avoid the dreaded C-Curve position while hitting your targets for the three exercise prongs. My meal plan will help you ditch the scale and see those beautiful abs you've already got. (Yes, you *do* already have them!)

Let's get started.

PART ONE

THE THEORY
WHY SIT-UPS ARE STUPID AND CRUNCHES ARE CRAP

■

1.

ABS: WHY WE WANT 'EM AND WHY WE NEED 'EM

I get it that you want to look good.
Feeling good is essential, too!

YOU CANNOT TURN on your television or go online without seeing ads for machines or training books that promise to give you "rock solid" abs. The pressure for everyday Americans to look beautiful and lean is everywhere. Most Americans are subsequently fed up with their bodies. According to research reported by Psych Central (2018), about 80 percent of American women are dissatisfied with their bodies.

I find a *Glamour* magazine study from 2011 particularly impactful, even today. They asked young women across the country to note every negative thought they had about their bodies over the course of one day, and 97 percent of the participants had at least one "I hate my body" moment. Men seem to report less on body image and there is more variation in statistics, but it's fair to say that a large number of men also feel negatively about their bodies.

The BuzzFeed Body Image Survey of 2014 allowed readers to say how they feel about their body and immediately see how others were answering the same question. Sixty-seven percent of responders either disliked or hated their stomach, whereas only 17 percent of responders liked or loved their stomach. According to research carried out by the University of the West of England in 2011, approximately a third of *all* undergraduates would sacrifice at least a year of their life for a "perfect" body.

Aesthetically, the stomach is one of the hardest parts of the body to hide and is the one area of the body that most people want to change. But getting a flat, firm stomach takes on a way more important role when you realize that your belly is an absolute vital sign in determining your health. Researchers followed about 360,000 Europeans who enrolled in one of the largest, longest health studies in the world and published their findings in the *New England Journal of Medicine* in November 2008. The report stated that *people with the most belly fat had about two times the risk of dying prematurely as people with the least amount of belly fat.*

Other than drinking or smoking, there aren't any simple individual characteristics that can increase a person's risk of premature death to this extent. Specifically, belly size is the leading predictor of heart disease, high blood pressure, and cholesterol, all of which can lead to heart attack and stroke. The study also concluded that people who were both obese and had a large belly were three times more likely to be diagnosed with dementia in later years than those of normal weight and belly size.

Research updated in *Harvard Health* in October 2015 and discussed in the *New York Times* in June 2018 explains that fat cells—particularly abdominal fat cells—are biologically active. In the *Times* article, titled "The Dangers of Belly Fat," Jane E. Brody details how visceral fat, which accumulates around abdominal organs, has been strongly linked to a host of serious disease risks, including heart disease, cancer, and dementia.

Harvard Health encouraged this fat to be thought of as an endocrine organ or gland, producing hormones and other substances that affect our health. Excess body fat, especially abdominal fat, disrupts the normal balance and functioning of these hormones. The *International Journal of Endocrinology* published a 2012 study titled "Androgens and Adipose Tissue in Males: A Complex and Reciprocal Interplay," which revealed how too much visceral abdominal fat appears to interfere with testosterone production and how low testosterone levels create even more abdominal fat. Scientists are also learning that visceral fat pumps out biochemicals that affect our immune system, which increases the risk of cardiovascular disease and has harmful effects on cells' sensitivity to insulin, blood pressure, and blood clotting.

Another reason excess visceral fat is so harmful could be its location near the portal vein, which carries blood from the intestinal area to the liver. When substances released by visceral fat, like free fatty acids, enter the portal vein and travel to the liver, they can increase the production of blood lipids in the bloodstream and raise your cholesterol levels. When you reduce your unhealthy fat intake, you not only tend to lose weight but also reduce your cholesterol levels.

Lastly, visceral fat is directly linked to insulin resistance, meaning that it can cause your body's muscle and liver cells to not respond adequately to normal levels of insulin. When glucose levels in the blood rise, your risk for diabetes increases.

All of this research proves that visceral abdominal fat actively affects various parts of your body and impacts your overall health. Considering that approximately 39 percent of adult Americans and 20 percent of American children are obese, we have to do something. Our desire for great-looking abs may be powerful, but our *need* for flatter stomachs is significant and cannot be overstated.

And if your increased risk of disease and death wasn't enough to convince you to flatten your stomach . . .

It is a fact that people with larger bellies have less sex (that decrease in testosterone described by the *International Journal of Endocrinology* study also decreases sex drive), have more anger, and suffer more from fatigue, depression, and sleep apnea.

It has been proven that people with larger bellies, especially women, unfortunately even make less money and have greater difficulty getting a job. Fairygodboss got a lot of buzz in 2017 with a survey of 500 hiring professionals about their biases when interviewing women. Twenty-one percent described the heaviest-looking women as "lazy" and "unprofessional." That description was selected less frequently for every

---

other kind of woman. Only 18 percent said the heaviest-looking woman had leadership potential, and only 15.6 percent said they would consider hiring her.

Scientists at the University of Exeter have found evidence that being a more overweight woman leads to lower opportunities in life, including lower income, which was corroborated by Jennifer Bennett Shinall, assistant professor of law at Vanderbilt University in Nashville, Tennessee, who reported on an "obesity wage penalty" for heavyset women compared with women of normal weight.

2.

THE ANATOMY OF THE ABS

OKAY, SO NOW you know that crunches cause excess flexion, and you understand the importance (not just the vanity) of maintaining a healthy waistline and why you can't just rely on your scale to tell you if you are healthy. Before we can fully dive into the theory of proper ab exercises, it's important to understand the anatomy of the abs.

The abdominal muscles consist of three muscle groups:

1. rectus abdominus: the front middle muscle, which runs from your ribs to your groin and contains the "six pack"
2. obliques: the side abdominal muscles, which run from your ribs down your sides to your hips
3. transversus abdominus: a small internal abdominal muscle

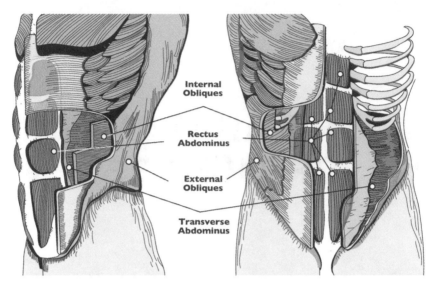

A view of abdominal muscles

It is vital to understand the far-reaching effects the abdominals can have. The abdominal muscles are required for lifting, running, walking, and even breathing.

The main muscle that everyone seems to concentrate on when they exercise is called the rectus abdominus. Its main purpose is to do flexion, the action of bringing your ribs closer to your groin. This is what you do for a sit-up or a crunch. Many people believe that this muscle actually strengthens and stabilizes their back, leading them to do more and more sit-ups and crunches.

A stable spine keeps you upright, helps you breathe properly, and makes your abdominals stronger. But this muscle has nothing to do with the stabilization of the spine—its only job is flexion or bending forward.

The obliques/side abdominal muscles (known as love handles or spare tires when we're out of shape) are broken down into two parts: internal obliques and external obliques. The job of these muscles is to connect the back muscles with the rectus abdominus, so that you can twist and rotate your body.

The muscle most often overlooked in the abdominal region, despite its prime importance, is the transversus abdominus. This deep underlying muscle has little to do with appearance but a lot to do with function. This is the muscle that stabilizes the spine and acts like an internal girdle, keeping organs from drooping or falling, which is important for optimal organ function.

It is important to work all three of these muscles—as well as to counteract all of the over-work they do, particularly the rectus abdominus.

This leads us to the topic of exercise and, again, the widespread belief that sit-ups and crunches are the best thing you can do to achieve an optimum waist measurement and six-pack abs. Even the exercise experts believe it.

Here's a patient story of an athlete who didn't see his training to be the cause of his pain at all. Dan Ownes didn't realize he was over-exercising and doing his core more harm than good!

ONE PATIENT'S STORY

MY NAME IS DAN OWNES, and I am a personal trainer and fitness model in New York City. While you may not know me, you may recognize my abs, which have been featured in hundreds of magazines and numerous books. My friends have called me "The Bod" because my face always seems to get cut out of the photos! I am telling you this to impress

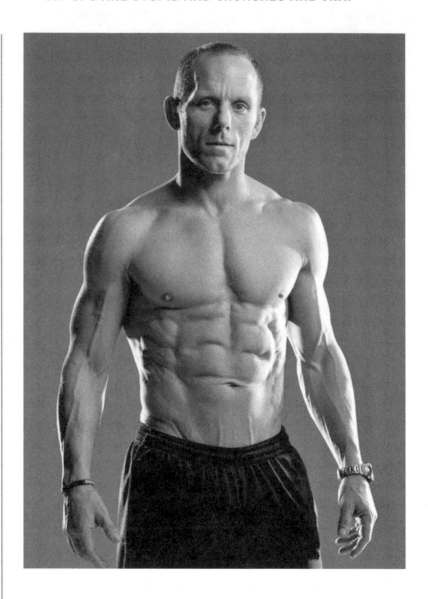

upon you that I was pretty sure that I knew it all when it came to core training. Heck, I am the core-training expert! People pay me hundreds, if not thousands, of dollars just so I can train them to get the great-looking abs that I have.

Well, this all changed after I hurt my neck. Being that I work out of a physical therapy center and gym, I consulted with the physical therapist about my neck pain, which was radiating into my shoulders. After months of treatment, I just couldn't get any relief. I was in severe pain, barely able to work, and training was downright impossible.

I went for a consultation with Dr. Sinett, and he discovered that my neck and shoulder pain was not coming from my neck or shoulders but rather from my imbalanced core. I couldn't believe what he was telling me. *How could I have an unbalanced core?*

Dr. Sinett added much-needed extension to my spine. He then told me that the source of my neck and shoulder pain was from my abdominals being shortened and over-contracted. Yes, they looked great, but they were too tight, throwing off the balance of the core. It was as if a straitjacket was pulling down my abs, resulting in tremendous pressure and pain in my neck and shoulders. In four visits, I was feeling 100 percent. My pain was gone, my strength was back, and I was changed forever.

The theory that sit-ups are stupid and crunches are crap is the most revolutionary concept that I have come across in the past twenty-two years of personal training. Not only will I never do a sit-up or crunch again, but I will never let any of my clients do them either. It is mind-boggling to me that something so simple can make such a huge difference.

—DAN OWNES

3.

THE BUSINESS OF ABS

S O, AMERICANS WANT good-looking abs, and experts believe crunches are the way to get them. Enter the Business of Abs.

Americans spend millions upon millions of dollars on abdominal machines. My personal feeling is that most of them wind up becoming expensive places to pile laundry. Then, why do they sell? Well, the manufacturers of these machines use professional fitness models with great-looking abs. They tell you that you, too, can have great abs if you just use their machines (even if their models have never used them).

Ultimately, the marketers of these machines base their advertising on a BS theory called "spot reducing." This is the practice of isolating a specific body part and exercising it with little regard for the rest of your body. You cannot take a specific body part and isolate that muscle to look great, yet these marketing misconceptions continue to be prevalent.

The reality is, you are either in shape or not. This is called the "all or nothing principle." Simply stated, you cannot have lean abdominal muscles and out-of-shape flabby arms. This is the reason all abdominal models look good all over, not just in their midsection: it's "all or nothing."

In fact, the abdominal machines do not make you leaner. The advertising pitch is similar to the sugary breakfast cereal pitch we all received as kids. The sugary cereals were *part* of a nutritious breakfast. However, they were *not* the nutritious part. Our nutrition from the breakfast came from the milk, fruit, juice, and even bacon that were put alongside the cereal bowl.

What most buyers are missing is the fine print that should be at the end of the commercial: these machines will not work without a proper diet. Abdominal machines are only part of a diet and exercise plan—and because they promote crunching, they are not the best way to exercise.

Spot reducing, the fine print . . . the Business of Abs is bogus for many reasons, but the biggest is this: crunch-based workouts disregard proper anatomy and physiology.

FUNCTIONAL INTERCONNECTEDNESS

Why are crunch-less workouts an appealing concept, and why are they starting to become more prevalent? It seems most people inherently either know sit-up exercises are wrong or have gotten injured doing them. While the people who have developed or touted crunch-less workouts do not necessarily understand why the injuries are occurring or why so many people have resisted doing sit-ups or crunches, they are filling a need.

The "why" for injuries lies in understanding our anatomy. As I have explained, harmful flexion exercises such as sit-ups and crunches can create much pain and many injuries throughout the body. Unfortunately, our society views our body as separate but connected pieces when it is actually one completely inter-woven whole. Essentially, every muscle and bone is related and affects all others.

In a book called *Anatomy Trains*, Thomas Myers uses the metaphor of railway or train lines to explain our functional anatomy as tissue trains that run throughout our body. Because we have myofascial meridians, or lines of pull, patterns of strain communicate through the myofascial "railroad," contributing to postural compensation and movement instability.

Because of the far-reaching functions of the abs and back, I call these two muscle groups "the superpowers." Their functions are very much linked, and their importance cannot be overstated. "There's so much mythology out there about the core," maintains Stuart McGill, a highly regarded professor of spine biomechanics at the University of Waterloo in Canada and a back-pain clinician. "The idea has reached trainers and through them the public that the core means only the abs. There's no science behind that idea."

The "core" remains a somewhat nebulous concept, but most researchers agree that it is the corset of muscles and connec-tive tissue that encircle and hold the spine in place. If your core is stable, your spine remains upright, while your body swivels around it. But, McGill says, the muscles forming the core must be balanced to allow the spine to bear large loads.

If you concentrate on strengthening only one set of muscles within the core, you can destabilize your spine by pulling it out of alignment. As for the abdominals, no sit-ups allowed, says McGill; they place devastating loads on the disks. "I see too many people who have six-pack abs and a ruined back," he concludes.

My patient Mo Auguste Maurepaz, "The Mambo-Kid" and a world super middleweight kickboxing champion, allowed me to see McGill's theory come to life. Mo came to my office to get help with his aching back and shoulders. As a professional fighter, Mo just thought that the aching was his "normal." I examined him and found some significant weaknesses throughout his body and ultimately discovered that the cause of his pain and weakness was his core imbalance.

His reaction? "That's impossible! I do thousands of crunches and sit-ups a day. Every fighter does! The thought of a fighter not doing sit-ups and crunches is like a ballerina not stretching."

Yes, crunches and sit-ups *are* completely ingrained in all fighters' regimens, but I started to show him how wrong sit-

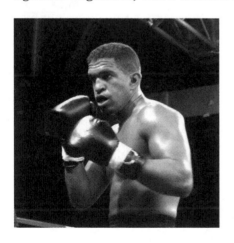

ups and crunches are and how much better his body would function by correcting his core imbalance. In just five minutes, Mo was convinced and cut out sit-ups and crunches, replacing them with both the core-strengthening and extension exercises provided in Part Two of this book. Now, he says he feels twenty years younger, and his results in the ring have shown it.

So, an imbalance in one area can create not only a cascade of imbalances throughout the body but can also be the cause of any injury. The term I use to describe this theory is *functional interconnectedness.*

We see this come into play in even the slightest of injuries, like an ankle twist. When you start to alter your normal walking mechanisms to accommodate the sore ankle, all of a sudden knee pain and low back pain are not far behind. It's not just your ankle that is affected but your entire body's function.

While this concept is common sense, I still receive bewildered looks when I tell a patient that their headaches are coming from their crunch-filled abdominal workout or even that their knee pain or foot pain is due to their core imbalance. The misunderstanding of how all our anatomy is connected is at the crux of the problem, and our overspecialized medicine is missing the big picture with a myopic approach. Viewing our anatomy with a mind for functional interconnectedness allows us to recognize distant influences and teaches us how the body can be impacted and affected by them.

Here are some other "Whys?" that prove functional interconnectedness is real:

WHY BODYBUILDERS CANNOT TURN THEIR HEADS

The common misconception is that body builders' overdeveloped shoulders get in the way; this is why they cannot turn their heads. This is not the case—it's just not how the body is designed. A developed muscle in one area will not get in the way of another muscle's function.

Weight lifters have just spent so much time doing sit-ups and crunches that they have shortened the abdominals, increasing the downward pull on the neck and thus making it difficult to turn their heads.

WHY PREGNANT WOMEN GET BACK PAIN

Large belly size is a main reason why pregnant women suffer from back pain. As the baby and the mother's belly grow, this creates a larger pull forward. This forward pull or hunch destabilizes the core, resulting in pain not only in the lower back but also the neck and shoulders.

The lower back can get so thrown off that a pregnant woman (or any person with excess belly fat, for that matter) can suffer from a nerve irritation called sciatica, which is characterized by pain radiating down the legs. The standing abdominal stretch and the thumbs-to-pit stretches (pages 65-66) are great anti-flexion exercises for pregnant women, though all of the exercises in this book are safe for expectant mothers.

4.

THE CONCEPT OF REFERRED PAIN

The problem might not be where the pain is.
(Remember interconnectedness!)

F I WERE to tell you that the spine is a closed kinetic chain, you may say, "Huh?" The best way to describe it is this: If you took a shoelace and stapled the top and bottom of it to a piece of paper and then twisted the lower part of the shoelace, what do you think would happen to the rest of the shoelace? It would all get twisted. The shoelace is your spine.

So, what does this mean? Well, going back to functional interconnectedness, an injury or an imbalance in one place can trigger pain and discomfort someplace else entirely. In fact, frequently wherever the pain is, the problem isn't.

When we talk to patients about their back pain, we describe the pelvis as the foundation of the house, with the head, neck, and shoulders being the second floor. That song we all learned in kindergarten is true, but there's more to it: the foot bone is not just connected to the ankle bone; it's also connected to the knee bone, which is then connected to the thigh bone and then to the hip bone and every other bone in your body.

There are thousands of cases in our office where the patient complains of low back pain, and yet the problem is coming from their feet. I have also seen patients with shoulder pain, yet the problem comes from their neck. My patients Dan and Mo from earlier both complained of neck pain, even though the problem wasn't in their necks.

NON-CONTACT INJURIES: A PREVENTABLE EPIDEMIC

The sufferers go far beyond my patients. Athletes who should be examples of prime fitness are experiencing an epidemic of non-contact injuries. This is because our current training regimens have turned us into fit but unhealthy people with unbalanced biomechanics.

Results published in the *Epidemiology of Collegiate Injuries* reveal that non-contact injuries represent 36.8 percent of all injuries. Between 70–84 percent of all ACL tears are non-contact related, or approximately 200,000 athletic injuries per year. The findings went on to state that an intrinsic risk factor for non-contact ACL tears is decreased core strength and decreased proprioception, or balance.

Ever wonder how a professional baseball player can tear a hamstring just running to first base? Or a football player can tear their knee while making a cut? I have. How can an athlete so finely tuned break down in the simplest of movements? It is my belief that no simple movement was the causative factor but rather the proverbial straw that broke the camel's back.

The only thing random that the body reacts to is trauma or an outside event such as falling off your bike or getting tackled in football. Everything else builds little by little internally. The current training methods of sit-ups and crunches create core imbalance, which destabilizes your entire body, resulting in injury.

For instance, core imbalance can cause an elevation of one side of your pelvis, causing one leg to be shorter than the other or creating too much rounded posture in your upper extremity. Once this happens, undue pressure is put on your feet, knees, back, and shoulders, leading to the tearing of ligaments, tendons, muscles, and discs and to the breakdown of joints.

So, the truth is that there are no "freak injuries." Core imbalance is frequently the cause. Non-contact injuries are *not* normal, just unfortunately common.

If you restore your normal core balance and biomechanics, the likelihood of non-contact injury is dramatically reduced.

THE PEN TRICK

This one always works and never ceases to amaze as a way to prove how imbalance affects the whole body. Have someone stand up with their arms out to their sides. Try to gently but firmly push down the person's arm. Barring any shoulder or neck injury, the person should be able to hold their arm against your pressure.

Now, have them stand with a pen under one foot. Retest the strength. It will immediately weaken. Take the pen away, and the strength will immediately return.

While this may seem a bit mind-boggling, it is normal neurology and happens with everyone. The body always needs to be in balance. When you create an imbalance by standing on the pen, immediately all of your muscles will go weak because your body is no longer in balance. A similar neurologic response is removing our hand quickly when it touches a hot stove.

Just to recap, the whole body is related. When the body is in balance, it functions optimally. When it isn't in balance, it will break down. It is not a question of if but when.

5.

BUSTING THE ABS MYTHS

S WE ARE learning, there are lots of myths out there about the abs and how to train them. Here are my top 10 Abs Myths:

MYTH 1:
I HAVE A WEAK CORE THAT
NEEDS TO BE STRENGTHENED.

Truth: I cannot begin to tell you how many times a patient will tell me that they have a weak core. It is actually impossible to have a weak core. Your abs are continually contracted, shortened, and overworked from all of the forward posture of your daily life (like sitting at a computer all day). If you do improper training methods (like sit-ups and crunches), you further contract your core. The problem, then, is not that the core is weak but rather that it is imbalanced.

Think about it: our back and abs work together to compose the core. The core needs a balance between flexion and extension, or between forward bending and backward bending. If the back were the overworked muscle group or the core were weak in relation to the back, we'd be walking around in a back bend all day, looking like we were constantly dancing the Limbo. But we only go forward and consequently have a slumped, hunched posture. Our forward posture indicates that the abs are too strong for the back and are pulling the back into a forward lean, therefore throwing the core out of balance.

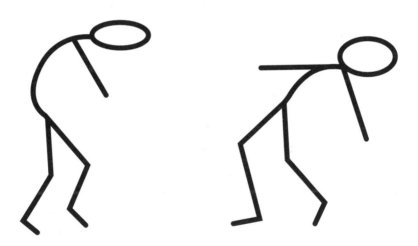

It's not that having strong abdominal muscles is bad; it's just that it is important to focus on strengthening the body as a whole rather than just one area. Most people's strength (or weakness) is relatively consistent throughout the entire body. In other words, one section is not significantly stronger or weaker than another.

Here's the bottom line: don't believe that your abs are the weakest part of your body. Yes, it's important to improve your physical function and strength but make sure to do so in a well-rounded way to achieve overall health.

MYTH 2:
LARGE AMOUNTS OF AB EXERCISES WILL GET RID OF MY GUT.

Truth: A landmark study at the University of Massachusetts found that large amounts of sit-ups or other abdominal exercises do not decrease the diameter of abdominal adipose cells (fat) or even abdominal circumference. So, you can't crunch your gut away.

As mentioned earlier, the common mistake in training is spot reducing. Working on one spot of your body simply doesn't work. If you really want the core of your dreams, you must practice my four-pronged approach, consisting of aerobic training, resistance/weight training, core training, and proper diet.

MYTH 3:
AN EXERCISE MAT AND BALL ARE THE BEST PIECES OF ABDOMINAL/CORE EQUIPMENT.

Truth: Actually the two best kinds of abdominal/core equipment are:

1. Your sneakers. They represent your ability to do cardiovascular exercise.
2. Your eating utensils: fork, knife, and spoon. You have to change your eating habits and replace unhealthy eating habits for healthier ones. In reality, you have to put down your silverware and eat a bit less if you want awesome-looking abs.

MYTH 4:
MY BIG GUT MEANS THAT I HAVE WEAK ABS.

Truth: This myth was best rebuked by a T-shirt that I once saw that said, "My beer gut is a protective layer of my six-pack abs." The big gut just represents a higher percentage of body fat. "But look at my flabby gut," patients will protest. "I can't have a strong core!"

If anything, the larger the gut, the more overworked the abs are; you are carrying around more weight on your front. Excess fat lies on top of the abs, and if your diet is poor, your flab will cover up the abs, making them look weak. Weak-looking abs do not indicate a weak core.

There are plenty of people who have big guts and really strong abs. I would never suggest that this guy has weak abs!

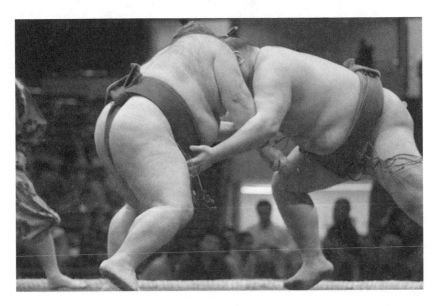

MYTH 5:
SIX-PACK ABS REPRESENT
GOOD ABDOMINAL TRAINING.

Truth: Just as we learned from Dan Ownes, six-pack abs don't represent good abdominal training. Six-pack abs just represent good-looking abs. In fact, six-pack abs probably represent an imbalanced core more than anything because most people who have six-pack abs have done a large number of sit-ups or crunches, or poor abdominal training.

MYTH 6:
GOOD FORM IS THE BEST WAY
TO PROTECT YOURSELF FROM INJURIES.

Truth: People hurt their necks from sit-ups and crunches not because of their form but rather because the exercise is simply harmful. If someone were to tug on the bottom of your shirt, you would feel the pull on your neck and shoulders. Sit-ups and crunches in any form create this same tugging, shortening your abs and pulling them, along with your neck and shoulders, into a harmful, curled C-like posture.

This C-like posture, which also compresses the spine, is what causes injuries, regardless of whether your hands support your neck or not. Supporting your head doesn't stop the damaging posture and therefore doesn't stop the pain and tension in your neck and shoulders.

MYTH 7:
CRUNCHES CAN HELP
STRENGTHEN MY BACK.

Truth: Crunches work the rectus abdominus, the function of which is forward bending, or flexion. This muscle has no stabilizing factor on the back. So, by crunching, you are actually working the wrong muscle for back stability. If you want to strengthen and balance your back, do an exercise called a skinny (see page 132), which works the transversus abdominus.

MYTH 8:
ABDOMINAL MACHINES ARE THE
SAFEST WAY TO WORK YOUR ABS.

Truth: Abdominal machines are probably the worst way to work your abs. Most of the abdominal exercise machines have isolated your abdominal muscles for more flexion (forward hunch), and we now know how bad that is for us.

MYTH 9:
PILATES IS A SAFE, LOW-IMPACT
WAY TO EXERCISE MY ABS.

Truth: Yes, it can be. The Pilates theory is to lengthen the core; I certainly subscribe to that theory. However, I've found that exercises like the Pilates 100 may put a person into excessive flexion. For Pilates to be effective, make sure you are doing, at a minimum, slightly more extension exercises than flexion. If you don't, injuries will occur.

MYTH 10:
LOW-FAT FOODS ARE VITAL FOR
GOOD-LOOKING ABS.

Truth: There are good fats, such as the ones found in avocados and olive oil, and bad fats, such as the ones found in chips and fast food. Eliminating good fats from your diets will not have a beneficial impact in your pursuit of six-pack abs. Eating right and reducing your portions is vital for getting six-pack abs. What we learned from my father's nine-month debilitating back pain is that, regardless of your weight, it is important to eat a good variety of healthy foods.

BONUS TRUTH: BETTER SEX

So, now you understand the myths and misconceptions created by The Business of Abs. Here's one extra perk about getting a balanced core (that The Business doesn't tell you): more and better sex! Here's why you should have it:

Improved sense of smell. After sex, production of the hormone prolactin surges. This, in turn, causes stem cells in the brain to develop new neurons in the brain's olfactory bulb, its smell center. Smell accounts for up to 90 percent of the way we taste food, so a better sense of smell lets us enjoy our meals more, sharpens our senses, and can improve our moods.

Weight loss, overall fitness. Sex, if nothing else, is exercise. A vigorous bout burns some 200 calories—about the same as running 15 minutes on a treadmill or playing a spirited game of squash. The pulse rate in an aroused person rises from about 70 beats per minute to 150, the same as that of an athlete putting forth maximum effort. Muscular contractions during sex work the pelvis, thighs, buttocks, arms, neck, and thorax.

Sex also boosts production of testosterone, which leads to stronger bones and muscles. A 2001 Queens University study even showed that by having sex three or more times a week, men reduced their risk of heart attack or stroke by half.

Pain relief. Immediately before orgasm, the hormone oxytocin surges to five times its normal level. This, in turn, releases endorphins, which alleviate the pain of everything from headaches—even migraines—to back pain and arthritis. In women, sex also prompts production of estrogen, which can reduce the pain of PMS.

Less-frequent colds and flus. Wilkes University in Pennsylvania in 2009 found that individuals who have sex once or twice a week show 30 percent higher levels of an antibody called immunoglobulin A, which is known to boost the immune system.

A happier prostate? Some urologists (most recently in a 2016 *European Eurology* study) believe they see a relationship between *in*frequency of ejaculation and cancer of the prostate. The causal argument goes like this: To produce seminal fluid, the prostate and the seminal vesicles take such substances from the blood as zinc, citric acid, and potassium, then concentrate them up to 600 times. Any carcinogens present in the blood likewise are concentrated. Rather than have concentrated carcinogens hanging around causing trouble, it's better to "evict" them.

6

FALSE INDICATORS OF HEALTH: BMI AND WEIGHT

ANOTHER FALSE BELIEF that many people incorrectly rely on is the idea that BMI and the scale can tell them if they are healthy. But these two abdominal health measurements are worthless. Here's why:

1.
BMI, OR BODY MASS INDEX (I LIKE TO CALL IT THE BAD MEASURING INDEX)

The equation for BMI, long considered the standard for measuring the amount of fat in a person's body, may not be as accurate as originally thought, according to new research published in March 2019 in *Medicine & Science in Sports & Exercise*, the official journal of the American College of Sports Medicine. BMI is determined by this mathematical formula: a person's weight is divided by his or her height in inches squared. Generally a BMI of 25 or above indicates a person is overweight; 30 or above indicates obesity. A person with a higher BMI is thought to be at a greater risk of heart disease, diabetes, and other weight-related problems.

The research team from Michigan State University and Saginaw Valley State University that helmed the latest study measured the BMI of more than 400 college students, some of them athletes and some not. In most cases, the student's BMI did not accurately reflect his or her percentage of body fat.

The BMI formula cannot be accurately used as a way to determine abdominal health because it doesn't address the different types of body makeup, gender, age, or how muscular a person is. This is especially true when BMI is used to measure athletes: a large percentage of them are often considered to be obese, according to their BMI, when in fact they are not. Many athletes tend to have a high BMI due to muscle mass, not due to body fat.

If BMI cannot accurately differentiate between muscle and fat, then how do we know whether one has too much body fat or muscle mass? A more accurate measurement is to look at body composition. Body composition is made up of total body water percentage, body fat, bone mass, and muscle fat. *Medical News Today* also suggested in August 2017 that Waist to Height Ratio or BMI with waist circumference provides a more accurate measure.

2.
SCALES

People have a strange fascination with scales and subsequently with their weight. Some people will stand on the scale every day as part of their daily ritual. Other people make it their business never to step on the scale, displaying almost a phobia about their overall weight.

Weight loss is a multibillion-dollar industry that has even spilled into the entertainment industry, with shows like *The Biggest Loser*, in which the contestant who loses the most weight wins. It seems that just about everyone is on a diet, all to accomplish one thing: "lose weight."

But even the research and data prove that diets don't work and that very few people ever stick to them. The *Washington Post* reported in January 2019 that 45 million Americans go on a diet each year, but only about 5 percent of dieters manage to keep the weight off long term. With 70 percent of US adults being overweight or obese, it's important to realize that scales and your overall weight are a misleading barometer of health and appearance. By setting up your goal to lose weight, you may be essentially missing the bigger picture and setting yourself up for failure.

Compare a 200-pound person with 7 percent body fat with a 200-pound person with 35 percent body fat. These two people weigh the same but will look very different. It's all about the percentage of your body fat in relation to your percentage of muscle.

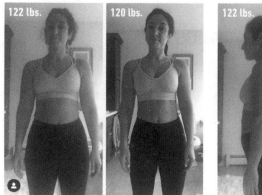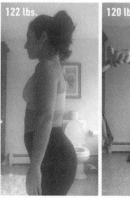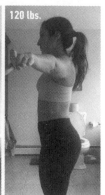

Elissa Parillo before and after she participated in a strength training program and clean eating plan. She never saw a big difference on the scale but did see a difference in the appearance of her body, as well as in her energy levels and self-satisfaction!

Which weighs more, muscle or fat?

This question reminds me of a riddle that I ask my kids: Which weighs more, a pound of rocks or a pound of feathers? The answer is that they weigh the same, one pound. However, the difference is the volume. A pound of feathers is a lot bulkier than a pound of rocks. One pound of fat takes up 18 percent more space than a pound of muscle.

So, what does this have to do with weight loss?

One pound of muscle has a lot less volume than one pound of fat. Once a person starts to exercise, they will increase their muscle percentage while subsequently decreasing their fat percentage. The results on the scale at this time could be downright depressing because your weight could stay the same or even go up. People who don't understand this concept may get frustrated in their pursuit of weight loss and give up, rather than continuing to work to make their body healthier and physically more appealing.

■

TWO WAYS TO ACCURATELY DETERMINE YOUR ABDOMINAL HEALTH

There are only two accurate ways to measure your abdominal health:

1. Percentage of body fat
2. Waist size

PERCENTAGE OF BODY FAT

Instead of weight loss, focus on your inches and how your clothes fit. By getting into shape, your body will have less volume. If you really want to pay attention, buy a body fat composition machine, which measures your percentage of body fat. These relatively inexpensive machines can electronically measure your percentage of fat to muscle. This whole process just takes a little more patience because the percentage of change is slower.

What follows are the normal and abnormal ranges of percentages of fat. Women tend to have a more difficult time achieving six-pack abs because their bodies require a higher percentage of body fat.

Women

AGE	UNDER FAT	HEALTHY RANGE	OVERWEIGHT	OBESE
20–40 yrs.	Under 21 percent	21–33 percent	33–39 percent	Over 39 percent
41–60 yrs.	Under 23 percent	23–35 percent	35–40 percent	Over 40 percent
61–79 yrs.	Under 24 percent	24–36 percent	36–42 percent	Over 42 percent

Men

AGE	UNDER FAT	HEALTHY RANGE	OVERWEIGHT	OBESE
20–40 yrs.	Under 8 percent	8–19 percent	19–25 percent	Over 25 percent
41–60 yrs.	Under 11 percent	11–22 percent	22–27 percent	Over 27 percent
61–79 yrs.	Under 13 percent	13–25 percent	25–30 percent	Over 30 percent

WAIST SIZE

"In addition to the stethoscope around their necks, physicians should be carrying a tape measure," Tobias Pischon, MD, said in the November 2012 issue of the *New England Journal of Medicine*. There is no need for the high-tech solution. The measurement is simple: if you want great-looking, thin abs, you need a waist size of 35 inches or less for men and 34 inches or less for women, with adjustments of course for individual body frames. Yes, there is the odd exception, but for the most part, the pelvic anatomy should take up this amount of space; otherwise the rest is just fat.

If you are a male and currently have a 38-inch waist, you are going to need to drop at least three inches off of your waist if you have any hope of getting six-pack abs. Of course, no abdominal product manufacturer wants to tell you this because it would severely reduce their clientele.

Measuring waist circumference is a more accurate predictor of visceral fat than body mass index. Researchers have found a direct correlation between waist size and risk of diabetes and heart disease (American Heart Association, 2007). By getting into shape, your body will have less volume.

Simply put, if you want six-pack abs, your waist size needs to be 35 inches or below.

7.

DON'T FORGET ABOUT POSTURE: YOUR CORE DEPENDS ON IT

PEOPLE WANT GOOD posture, but very few people even know what having good posture means. Posture plays a much more important role than just looking taller. As we now know, a spine out of normal alignment is susceptible to injury, so good health is impossible to achieve without good posture.

■

PERSONAL POSTURE ASSESSMENT

Your mother continually telling you not to slouch or to sit up straight can't fix posture. So how do you assess your posture? Stand in front of a mirror and check yourself out.

Facing front, answer these questions without adjusting your natural posture:

Is your head held straight and eyes level?

Is your chin straight?

Are your shoulders even?

Are your hips level?

Do your arms hang in front of you with your thumbs facing out?

Do your knees face straight ahead?

Are your feet straight?

Now turn toward your side.

Does your ear line up with your shoulder?

Does your shoulder line up with your hips?

Do your hips line up with your knees and ankles?

If you answered no to any of the above questions, your posture is not ideal. You likely have core imbalance and are compromising your body by placing undue pressure on it.

For example, thumbs that rotate inward lead to rounded shoulders and an internally rotated chest muscle. If your feet aren't straight, unnecessary pressure is put not only on your feet but also on your knees, which alters your gait, affecting the whole interconnected muscle railroad of your body.

COMPRESSION VS. EXPANSION

Poor neck posture generally causes your neck to go too far forward. For every inch that your head moves forward, the weight of your head on the neck and shoulders increases by 10 pounds. This extra pressure on the neck reduces the normal curvature of the cervical, or neck and spine, resulting in strained muscles, ligaments, bones, and joints or even in arthritis when those joints break down from the pressure. The end result is either acute or chronic pain.

Your middle back is known as the thoracic spine, which has a normal curve called a kyphosis. When we have too much of a forward hunch, typically more than 35 degrees, this is called a hyper-kyphosis. This hunch means forward-rounded shoulders and head posture, which adds a compressive load on the spine.

Prolonged sitting in front of computers is just one of the factors contributing to the misalignment of the spine and increased kyphosis. The vast majority of the population is doing way too much sitting and expresses way too much forward posture. Many of us are, indeed, suffering from hyper-kyphosis.

When your spine is hunched forward or compressed, you have decreased flexibility, decreased blood flow, decreased lymph drainage, decreased oxygen intake, and impaired health. On the other hand, when you have spine and chest expansion, you have increased flexibility, increased blood flow, increased lymph drainage, increased oxygen intake, and thus better health.

In Aruba, the wind only blows in one direction so much that the native Divi-divi trees literally grow bent over to one side.

With all of our forward hunching, we are starting to look like Divi-divi trees.

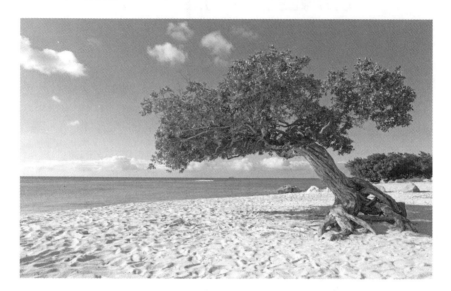

SITTING UP STRAIGHT MAY NOT BE THE ANSWER

While the worst posture that researchers have found is slouching forward, according to recent studies, sitting up straight also might not be a good thing. Utilizing MRI studies as well as evaluating compressive loads, researchers in 2006 found that sitting up straight keeps your spine at a 90-degree angle, which puts too much of a compressive strain on the body.

It was determined during this study that a 135-degree angle alleviated much of the compressive load (*Science Daily*). To achieve a 135-degree angle, sit with your feet on the floor and angle your torso back. By leaning back in your chair, you are opening the space in your chest as well as relaxing your musculature. While this may not be practical for doing computer work, anytime you have the ability to lean back in your chair (while on the phone or reading, for example), you should do so. Recline your seat back in your car a bit as well.

8

HEALING
YOUR CORE

POSTURAL IMBALANCE CAUSED by too much flexion also affects your internal organs and your ability to breathe properly. This really isn't a test but rather a way to illustrate that when your posture is open, your ability to breathe and take in more oxygen is much greater than when you are slouched forward and in a closed posture. In order to see how postural imbalance is affecting your ability to breathe properly, take this Deep Breath Test:

1. Stand with your arms turned in at your sides.
2. Take a deep breath.
3. Stand with your arms outstretched.
4. Take a deep breath.

Do you breathe better when you stand with your body more open? We all should. Breathing supplies our bodies and its various organs with the needed supply of oxygen and is also one means to get rid of waste products and toxins from the body.

The brain requires more oxygen than any other organ. If it doesn't get enough, the result is mental sluggishness, negative thoughts, depression, and, eventually, vision and hearing decline. The quickest and most effective way to purify the bloodstream is by taking in extra supplies of oxygen from the air we breathe. With better posture, you get a more open chest and more oxygen, benefitting every part of the body.

FIGHTING FLEXION

Other than leaning back in your chair when you can, how do you work against flexion? While you can stop crunching, you can't quit your desk job or cut out your commute. Here are two anti-flexion stretches that you can work into your daily routine.

THUMBS-TO-PITS STRETCH

■

Place your thumbs under your armpits with your fingertips pointed up to the ceiling. Now, tilt your head back and lift your thumbs up as high as possible. This stretch will open the chest and extend your mid-back.

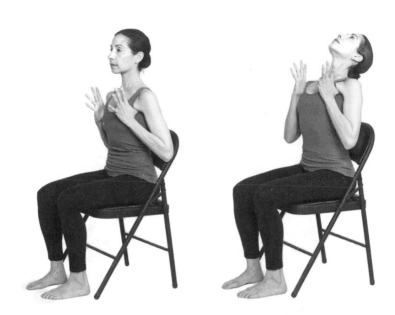

THE STANDING ABDOMINAL STRETCH

■

This stretch is a great way to make sure that you have the proper balance between flexion and extension. It can be done anywhere and takes just seconds to do. Stand up, raise your arms above your head, and lean your torso backward. I recommend doing this stretch 15 times every hour to my patients.

Do not go too far back—about a 30-degree angle will suffice. You should never feel pain while doing this. These stretches will relieve muscle soreness and tightness in your back, as well as dramatically improve your breathing.

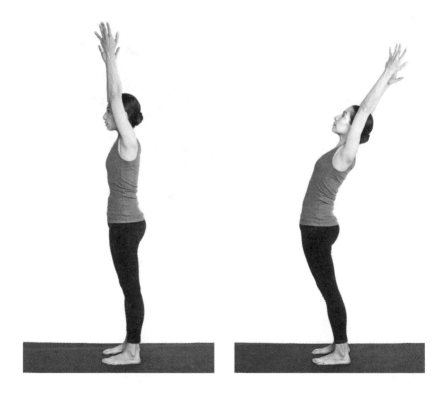

9

THE BACKBRIDGE BREAKTHROUGH

HEALING YOUR CORE IN
TWO MINUTES A DAY

AFTER MY DAD tried an extension on the exercise ball and promptly fell off, I knew back pain patients needed something with stability to help heal their core. I designed the Backbridge specifically to relieve core imbalance and subsequent back pain, as well as to increase flexibility and deep breathing by opening up the chest while correcting your posture.

As we have learned, the body derives its healing power from anatomical interconnectedness. The Backbridge helps to achieve a balanced core and therefore a sound body as a whole. Just think of the Backbridge as Invisalign® for your spine. It adds progressive extension to your body by gently fixing your spinal alignment and posture.

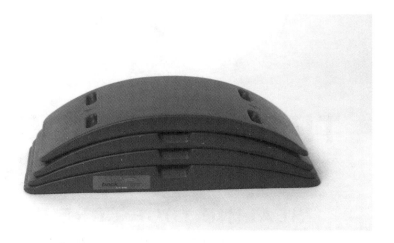

As we age, we lose the type of flexibility we enjoyed as children. And indeed, because of their limberness, children can use all five levels of the Backbridge with absolutely no problems. By using the Backbridge, you can effectively rediscover the limberness that you had as a child in a healthy, productive way.

Here's the story of one of my patients who also happened to be a famous athlete. Curing his core imbalance with Backbridge also turned out to be the cure for a host of non-contact injuries throughout his body:

ONE PATIENT'S STORY

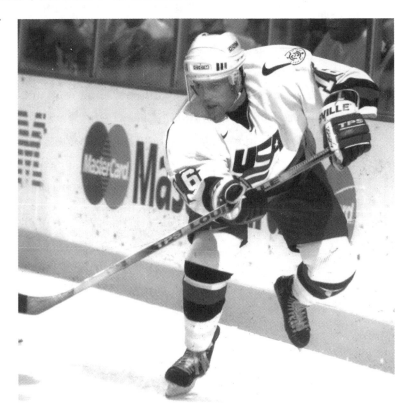

SINCE RETIRING FROM HOCKEY, I was suffering from tension in my jaw, neck, and shoulders, as well as a lot of foot and knee pain—to the point where I could barely exercise. Running was just out of the question.

I had reconstructive knee surgery when I was playing [hockey] and also dealt with numerous concussions. As a professional athlete, I had conditioned my body to continue to power through things; in my retirement years, I was struggling with a myriad symptoms. I was referred to Dr. Sinett by a colleague, and after examining me, he noticed that a lot of my symptoms were brought on by my forward hunched posture.

Dr. Sinett explained that I had spent more than thirty years bent over a hockey stick and that I needed to correct the effects. He prescribed me his Backbridge, and the results have been quite remarkable. Gradually, after using the Backbridge, my posture started to change, as did my suffering.

I am now exercising—even running—and feeling a ton better. I would recommend the Backbridge to anyone and would strongly insist any hockey players to make it part of their daily routine. This was something so simple but so profound for me!

—NHL HALL OF FAMER PAT LAFONTAINE

Remember how Dan Ownes was cured in just four visits? The Backbridge was what I used to put extension into his spine. Within two minutes of lying on the Backbridge, he felt considerably better. Two minutes after all of that pain and suffering is really all it takes to start the healing, and it's all it takes to keep you feeling good daily.

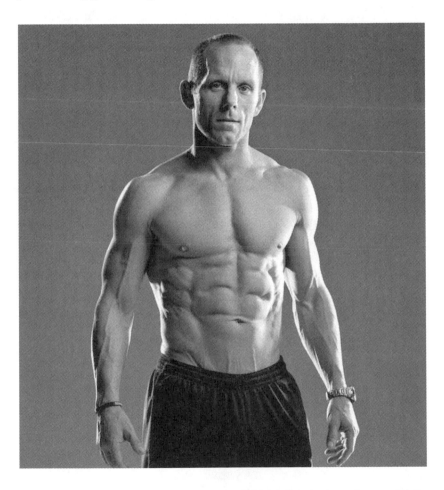

Abs this good-looking deserve to be included twice. And you know what?
Even after Dan Ownes ditched the sit-ups and the crunches,
he *still* looked this good.

DESIGN AND FEATURES OF THE BACKBRIDGE

The Backbridge's patented design consists of five height levels: the base level is 2 inches and the next four levels add 1.25 inches each, bringing the arch to 7 inches at its highest. Its stackable pieces allow users to take advantage of the level that best fits their needs—and store the remaining pieces until they progress. The ability to easily change the Backbridge height allows for quick adjustment of the degree of difficulty when integrating it into exercise, yoga, or stretching.

HOW TO USE THE BACKBRIDGE

The Backbridge is therapeutic as well as diagnostic. It is therapeutic because it will help you feel better and diagnostic because it evaluates how tight your spine really is. The Backbridge is recommended by therapists to help correct postural imbalance in their patients and to alleviate aches and pains. Lying over the Backbridge for just a few minutes a day will:

- relieve back, neck, and shoulder pain
- help to correct and reverse years of postural imbalance
- improve flexibility
- improve breathing by opening up the chest

To use the Backbridge properly, you must lie on it for two minutes in the morning and two minutes in the evening. Consistency is key. Slouching will occur daily, and counteracting this flexion must also be part of your daily routine.

Before you begin to use the Backbridge, please consider the following:

- The highest point of the Backbridge should be between your shoulder blades. It should never hurt; it should feel like a good, solid stretch.
- Your arms should be placed flat on the floor straight above your head for the maximum stretch. If that position is uncomfortable, you can fold your arms across your chest. It is always about comfort. I even have patients who feel most comfortable with their arms by their sides, in goal-post position or in a wide V. Find which position works best for you.

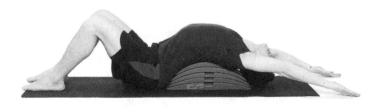

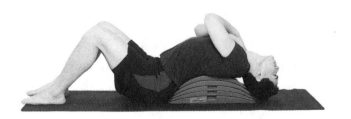

- Since comfort is the key to proper use of the Backbridge, you can put a rolled-up towel or a pillow under your knees if that helps you to have a more comfortable stretch. This may not be necessary for you, but for some people, it's helpful.
- If your neck or head is uncomfortable while lying on the Backbridge, put a pillow behind your head or even take the unused levels of the Backbridge and use them as a pillow.

For the Backbridge to be an effective tool in helping to ease your back pain, you must determine the best starting level for you and increase the levels as your body acclimates to each level. It doesn't matter where you start, it's where you get to—and it's not about ego.

The following guidelines will help you to determine where to start:

- Level 1 (2 inches): for people with significant back pain or the elderly with very limited flexibility
- Level 2 (3.25 inches): the most popular level, it is for people who are experiencing some back pain or discomfort but have fair to good flexibility
- Level 3 (4.5 inches): designed for healthy, active people
- Level 4 (5.75 inches): for those who are quite flexible and in very good physical shape
- Level 5 (7 inches): the highest level of usage for the Backbridge and designed for someone with excellent spinal flexibility, like a well-trained (read: core-

conscious) athlete or someone who has used the
Backbridge consistently for some time

Note: If you can't lie on the floor with Level 1, just use it on a
chair as a back support or lie on it on your bed. While the stretch
might not be as effective, it is a good way to start improving your
back flexibility. After a week or two of using it as a chair support,
try again with Level 1 on the floor and see if you are able to do it.
It's all about slow evolution and naturally easing your body in.

FREQUENTLY ASKED QUESTIONS ABOUT THE BACKBRIDGE

Who can use the Backbridge?

Just about everyone: kids, the elderly, pregnant women, and
the overweight included. While no product is appropriate for
everyone, the Backbridge comes pretty close.

*How long should it take to progress to a different level of the
Backbridge?*

Again, this process is unique to everyone, but as a general rule,
you should progress to the next level about every three weeks
(remember, this is if you are consistent with twice-daily use).
As mentioned, the most important aspect is comfort. When
increasing to a new level, do so for 30 seconds and then go
back and forth to your usual level, slowly adding more time to
the higher level.

The goal is not to get to the highest level but to improve

your flexibility, at the level best suited to your needs. If you find that you are using the Backbridge consistently for three weeks and are unable to progress, don't get discouraged. The Backbridge is still providing you with extension relief from the day's flexion, which will help you achieve core balance and back comfort, even without progressing quickly.

How do I get up after using the Backbridge?

It is very important to get up slowly by rolling to your side first, sitting up slowly, and then taking your time to get to your feet. You may get dizzy if you get up too fast from an arched position, so always remember to take your time.

How long should I use the Backbridge each time?

Use the Backbridge for two minutes in the morning and two minutes in the evening every day to counteract the flexion you do between those hours. Using the Backbridge consistently, day in and day out, will bring you the relief from back pain you are experiencing.

Should I sleep on the Backbridge?

No, I do not recommend sleeping on the Backbridge. Two minutes twice a day is plenty.

Is it possible to use the Backbridge in a sitting position? Do you still get the benefit from using it?

Absolutely. The Backbridge can provide relief when you must sit for long periods of time. You must first choose the correct level to properly support your back while sitting; the convex design will provide the necessary support to improve your posture and your back pain.

You can use the strap included when you purchase the Backbridge to securely attach it to your desk chair or even your car seat. The Backbridge is the only ergonomic chair device that supports your entire spine while allowing it the proper extension.

STRETCHING AND EXERCISE WITH THE BACKBRIDGE

When used for yoga, Pilates, abdominal exercises, strength training, or stretching, the Backbridge enables you to isolate movements, effectively allowing you to target certain areas and see the results you hope to accomplish.

Personal trainers, Pilates instructors, and yoga teachers have begun using the Backbridge in their fitness routines and are recommending this multipurpose device to their clients. Here's how they are using it:

- **Pilates:** As a barrel alternative, the Backbridge is more customizable and less expensive.

- **Yoga:** As a replacement for traditional yoga blocks, the Backbridge allows for contoured support and more versatility.

- **Stretching and Abdominal Work:** A safe alternative to an exercise-ball balance workout, the Backbridge is compact and easily adjusts for various levels of stretching and targeted abdominal work.

- **Strength Training:** The Backbridge is an assistance prop to support more than 100 different positions.

My book *The Ultimate Backbridge Stretch Book* is a great guide to integrating the Backbridge into your workouts. The Backbridge is an unbelievable piece of fitness equipment. It isolates your abdominal muscles, allowing you to get a great ab workout in about half the time. Its stackable components allow you to make exercises either easier or harder by altering the height. When you alter the height of the Backbridge, you are essentially able to raise or lower the floor, resulting in shorter or longer range of motion throughout the exercise.

Other than just lying on the Backbridge the regular way, here is one of my favorite stretches that is great to do before you start the exercise portion of this book. This stretch will loosen up your side muscles (latissimus dorsi) and stretch out your chest or pectoral muscles. You can even stretch your arms out to the sides and loosen up your chest muscles (pectoralis).

SIDE-LYING STRETCH

■

1. Lie on your side and stretch over the Backbridge so that it fits just above your hip.
2. Extend your top arm back for 10 seconds. As you progress, add more time and more levels of the Backbridge.
3. Switch sides and repeat.

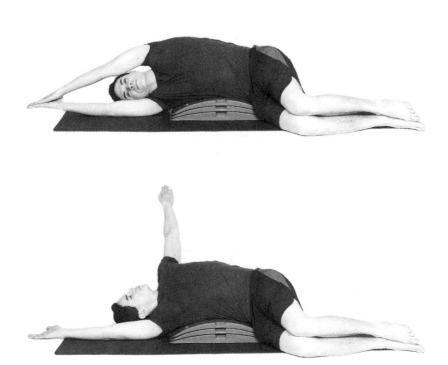

BACKBRIDGE TESTIMONIALS

"As a writer, sitting for extended periods of time—often hunched over my laptop—is an unfortunate reality of my daily life, and for a while, neck and back pain became an unfortunate reality as well. But thanks to Dr. Todd, it isn't anymore. The Backbridge has been crucial to helping me manage my neck and back problems."

—Keli Goff, author of *The GQ Candidate* and *Party Crashing*, and political commentator

"I was pregnant with twins and had been experiencing back pain since about week 8. I went to see Dr. Todd at 16 weeks, when it just got to be too much for me. After my first session with him, I purchased the Backbridge, and I haven't looked back. I lie on it every evening, and it has changed my life for the better."

—Heather Bostwick, mother of twins

"As a chiropractor, Dr. Sinett's Backbridge has been an invaluable tool in my office. The Backbridge is a groundbreaking product that addresses the most common of people's postural faults and corrects the problem quickly and painlessly."

—Dr. Peter Ottone, chiropractor

"The Backbridge has literally changed my life! I suffered with chronic low back pain for 23 years before I met Dr. Sinett. After a few short weeks, I was amazed at how much better I felt! Nothing helped until now. Thank you, Dr. Sinett, for changing my life!"

—Kevin Daily, hotel executive

"Since I started using the Backbridge, I've been able to release tension in my lower back, and it seems like I'm throwing my punches and kicks with more power and speed. It's like I'm 20 years old again."

—W.K.O. World Super-Middleweight Kickboxing Champion Maurepaz "The Mambo-Kid" Auguste

"After ten years or so of retiring from the NHL, my body started to come unhinged. I struggled with everything, from neck, jaw and shoulder tension to foot and knee pain. Dr. Sinett was the only physician who told me my pain was from 30 years of being bent over a hockey stick! He taught me how to correct the effects of too much forward hunch and helped me feel great again. His solution for reversing a hunched posture was simple but changed my life!"

—Pat LaFontaine, former NHL Hockey Player

PART TWO

NO PAIN, BIG GAIN!

THE FLAT ABS SOLUTION: THE SINETT EXERCISE AND NUTRITION COMBINATION

10.

THE NO-CRUNCH CORE PLAN

O N THE ONE hand, proper exercise is one of the most important things that you can do for your health, and it's critical to thrive in, not just survive, exercise. On the other hand, plenty of people are participating in exercise routines that are negatively affecting them.

Here are a couple of questions to ask yourself to determine if you are getting proper, healthy exercise:

Are you creating more hurt and harm by exercising?

As a person who consistently exercises, I have come to witness and read about exercise practices that are downright harmful. Dangerous exercise practices currently in vogue include: overtraining; elevating your heart rate too high; participating in too many long endurance races, like marathons, that break down your body; raising your speed, workout intensity, distance, or exercise time too quickly; and doing crunches and sit-ups.

These practices are leading people to increasingly reach for anti-inflammatories. Over-the-counter medications, such as Tylenol, Motrin, and Aleve, are more and more popular, and doctors at alarming rates are prescribing anti-inflammatories. There are also more and more orthopedic surgeries and joint replacements happening each year.

Take inventory of your body and your aches and pains, as well as your medicine cabinet, when answering this question.

Do you feel energized and loose after exercise or wiped out and exhausted?

If you feel wiped out after your exercise, it is unhealthy. Do you take Advil or Tylenol before or after you exercise? If so, there is something wrong, and your body is likely suffering the effects of inflammation and irritation. Are you exercising but hating every moment of it? If so, it is emotionally unhealthy. But instead of ditching exercise altogether, let's try to find a type of exercise that you enjoy and find fun. Dance in your living room to the radio, walk while listening to music, exercise in front of the television. Exercise is too important not to do, but make sure you are in tune with your body and aren't pushing yourself too far.

WHICH BRINGS US TO ABS . . .

"So how *can* I work out my abs?" is the question *every one* of my patients asks after I convince them how harmful sit-ups and crunches are. The question set me on a course to come up with a good answer.

Part One of this book was the why. Part Two is the how. My four-pronged No-Crunch Core Plan is the way to get the abdominals you always wanted without hurting yourself or doing sit-ups and crunches:

1. aerobic training
2. strength training
3. core and ab exercises
4. healthy eating

To do these things, you must have sneakers, a fork, willpower, patience, and persistence.

11.

AEROBIC EXERCISE

YOU CANNOT GET great-looking abdominals without being lean. As mentioned, strong abs can lie under fat—they just won't look great. Aerobic exercise is vital in obtaining a lean physique, which allows your six-pack to be seen.

Burn the calories, burn the fat, see the abs. You can dance it off, run or walk it off, but you must properly train your cardio-vascular system. Remember, slow and steady wins the race. Over-exertion or too much exercise is just as bad as not enough.

I have generally found that people who are doing aerobic exercise are overtraining themselves, thus making their bodies susceptible to injury. Aerobic-type classes can be dangerous because the instructor's heart rate is so much lower than the class participants, and therefore it can be hard for the instructor to gauge just how far they are pushing you. You must remember that you are only competing with yourself and not the person next to you, who might be in better aerobic shape. Enduring pain through a fitness class when your heart rate is too high is not the way to get into shape.

■

TRACK YOUR HEART RATE

With all of the wearable technology out there, I recommend that you track your heart rate when exercising. Before getting started with aerobic exercise, you must know your resting heart rate. Calculate your resting rate with your wearable technology or sit quite still before getting out of bed. Place the tips of your middle and index fingers on your wrist or neck right by your Adam's apple for a minute and count the beats. (Don't use your thumb because it has its own pulse.) Do this for five days and take the average.

A normal resting heart rate for adults ranges from 60 to 100 beats a minute. Generally, a lower heart rate at rest implies more efficient heart function and better cardiovascular fitness. For example, a well-trained athlete might have a normal resting heart rate closer to 40 beats a minute.

But, for the non-conditioned athlete, too low of a heart rate is called bradycardia. Low heart rates can be caused by disease or damage to the heart structure. An imbalance in electrolytes and some medications can also cause your pulse to drop.

Bradycardia is often diagnosed when the pulse drops below 60 beats per minute. If your pulse rate drops too low, you may feel light-headed, dizzy, faint, or very fatigued. If you have any of these symptoms, see your doctor. Bradycardia left untreated can lead to chest pain, high blood pressure, and even heart failure, and you should not begin aerobic exercise with this condition unless under the careful care of a physician.

◼

MY FIVE TIPS FOR LOWERING YOUR RESTING HEART RATE

1. Exercise. Light consistent aerobic exercise, such as walking, and some resistance training, like lifting light weights, will effectively lower your heart rate. (Overtraining can have the opposite effect.)

2. Avoid caffeine and alcohol.

3. Massage and acupuncture: A British study found that people who received an hour of reflexology once a week had rates that averaged eight beats per minute (BPM) lower.

4. Empty your bladder. Taiwanese researchers found that the stress of having a full bladder elevates the resting heart rate by an average of nine BPM.

5. Sleep more soundly, and reduce the noise. Each noise arousal spikes heart rates by an average of 13 BPM. Try a noise machine or ear plugs if you live in a city or elsewhere where you may be disrupted by noise.

CALCULATE YOUR MAX HEART RATE AND TRAINING RATES

You never want to exceed your maximum heart rate when training, but you can figure out how to train at different percentages of your max heart rate:

$$220 - \text{your age} = \text{maximum heart rate}$$

According to the American Heart Association, the target heart rate during exercise for most healthy people should range from 50 percent to 75 percent of your maximum heart rate. The more fit you are, the higher or harder you can train and the more you can increase your heart rate. The less fit you are, the lower you want to train.

For example, if you are a fit 40-year-old, you will base your training on: 220 - 40 = max heart rate of 180. Because you are fit, you can train up to 135 BPM, or 75 percent of the max heart rate of 180. Your target training zone would be from 125–135 BPM. For someone just getting into shape or recovering from an injury, it is recommended that you train at 50 percent of your max heart rate and slowly raise your target zone every few weeks. In the end, good, healthy exercise is all about safety.

THE RIGHT AMOUNT OF AEROBIC EXERCISE

People should perform aerobic exercise approximately four times a week for a minimum of 45 minutes. These 45 minutes should be broken down into three parts:

1. a 15-minute warm-up
2. a 15-minute training session within your target heart rate
3. a 15-minute cooldown

After these 45 minutes, you should feel refreshed and energized, not wiped out and exhausted. As you progress over time, you will notice improvements in your stamina.

RUNNING VS. WALKING

I like walking! Some people don't consider it to be a good workout, but it is lower impact than running, and you can get your heart rate up to training levels just by walking briskly. Walking is something that just about anyone can do. It is stress-reducing and can be done anywhere. You don't need special equipment, and walking will create the least amount of injuries, so get walking, people!

AVOID BIKING

While I applaud people who do cardiovascular exercise, you want to avoid exercises that will put your spine into a curled C-like pattern, such as cycling. Again, the simple theory is that we spend way too much of our day forward hunched, so choosing an exercise that brings more forward hunch just creates more imbalance. You can excercise before and after you ride or make sure that you are doing more of the anti-flexion exercises, such as thumbs-to-pits and standing abdominal stretches, throughout the day following a ride.

12.

STRENGTH TRAINING

STRENGTH TRAINING IS the next prong in our four-pronged approach to flat, healthy abs. When you do resistance training, you are creating tiny tears in your muscle fibers. From these tears, the body repairs itself, and the muscle structurally adapts. The muscle becomes stronger and more resistant to fatigue.

This process is called the training effect. It improves your muscle function and just about all aspects of your health. Resistance training makes your body burn more calories by speeding up your metabolism.

University of South Carolina researchers found that muscular strength can also improve your life expectancy. By improving your strength with resistance training, weight training, or even something as simple as push-ups, you can increase bone density, decrease your blood pressure, decrease your risk of stroke, cancer, and cardiovascular disease, and improve your ability to sleep, think, be happier, and reduce your stress. Even 30 minutes of resistance training a week decreases your risk of heart disease by 23 percent, according to a Harvard study.

It is never too late to start. People in their 80s have improved muscular strength by doing any form of resistance training.

Resistance training at any age should be done at least three days a week. Whether you join a gym to pump some iron, use resistance bands, or just use your body weight as your resistance and work out at home, I urge you to pick a routine that works for you and your time schedule. You want to do resistance training for the rest of your life, so set up a realistic routine for your schedule.

STRENGTH TRAINING WORKOUT

I have created a full-body fit band workout that is geared to people who want to get in shape at home or on the run in a manageable amount of time. Resistance training can be done anywhere with easy-to-transport resistance bands. The bands come in different colors to represent different resistance levels. If you find you need even more resistance, you can double up on band.

FRONT LATERAL PULL-DOWNS

■

With your hands shoulder-width apart, gripping the band, extend your arms at an angle above your head. Now, pull the band apart and lower your arms toward your chest. Release resistance and return arms to starting position. Repeat 12–15 times.

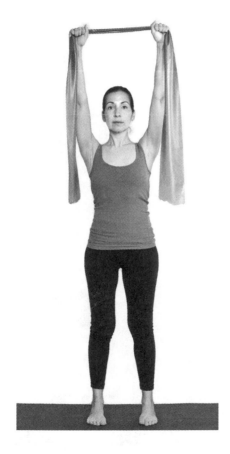
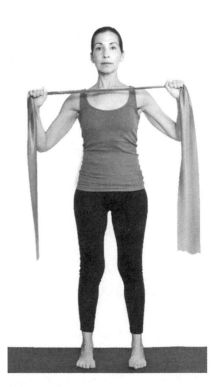

CHEST PRESS

■

Wrap the band behind your back at shoulder height. Grasp the band with your upper arms at your sides and elbows bent at a 90-degree angle. Slowly straighten your arms forward. Return to beginning position. Repeat 12–15 times.

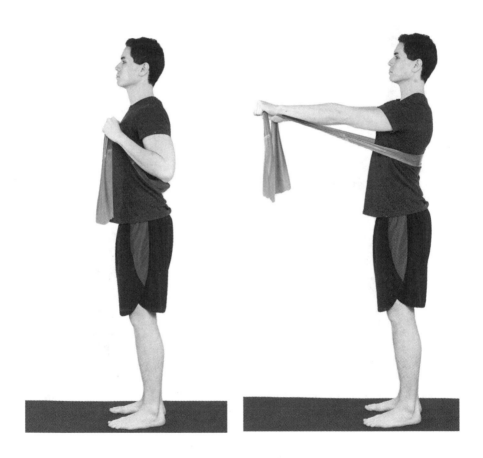

HUG THE TREE

■

Start in the same position as the chest press but with arms extended out to your sides and elbows slightly bent. Bring your arms forward until both fists touch in front of you (as if you were wrapping your arms around a tree). Return to starting position. Repeat 12–15 times.

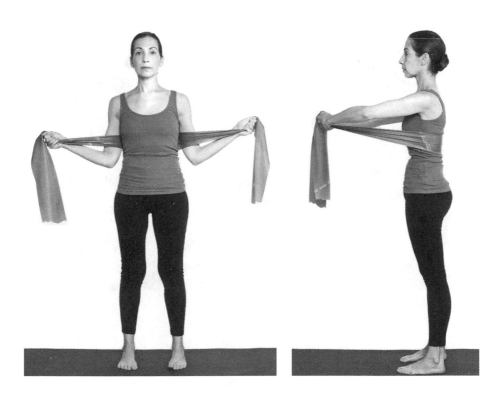

SHOULDER SHRUGS WITH SQUAT

■

Stand on the band, knees slightly bent. Grasping the band with hands beside your thighs, shrug your shoulders up toward your ears. Hold for count of three and release. Then, squat with a straight back, lowering your buttocks toward the floor. Return to standing and repeat.

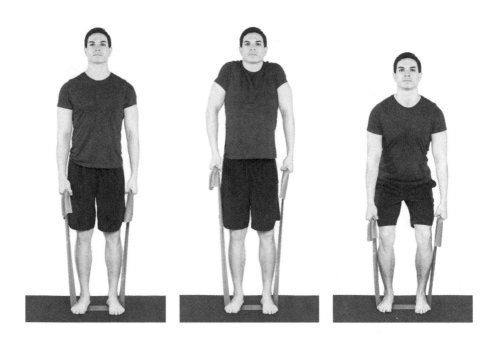

LATERAL RAISES

■

Stand on one end of the band with knees slightly bent. Grasp the other end of the band in your hand and raise your arm out to the side until it reaches shoulder height. Slowly return your hand to the side. Repeat 12 times and switch arms.

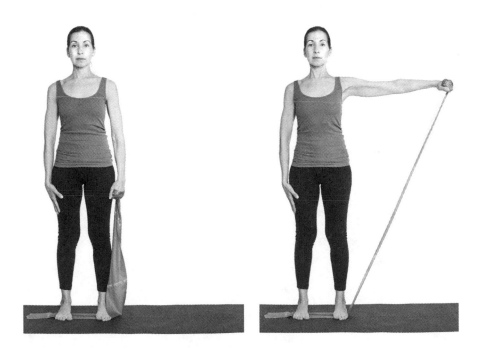

SHOULDER PRESS

■

Sit in a comfortable, cross-legged position on the band. Grasp the band and raise your arms to shoulder height, bending at the elbows in a goal-post position. Slowly straighten your arms above your head and bring your hands toward each other. Release back to starting position and repeat 12–15 times.

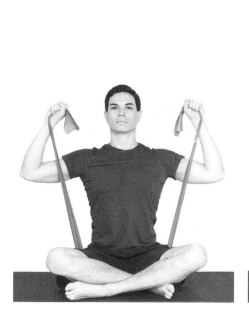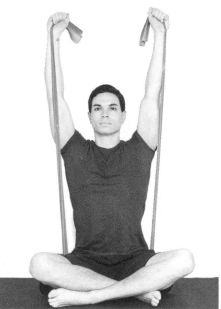

TRICEPS EXTENSION

■

Standing on the band, bend forward at the hips with knees
slightly bent. Grasp the band in both hands with elbows bent
and arms close to your sides. Slowly extend your arms straight
back and up behind you. Do 12 repetitions.

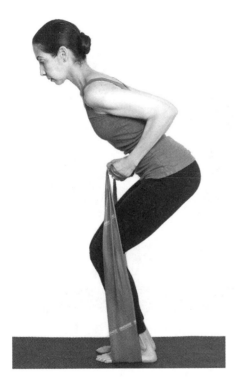
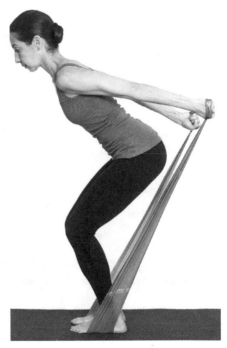

PULL-APARTS

◼

Grip the band behind you with straight arms, palms facing back. Slowly pull hands away from each other, increasing tension on the band. Hold for three seconds and return to starting position. Repeat 12–15 times.

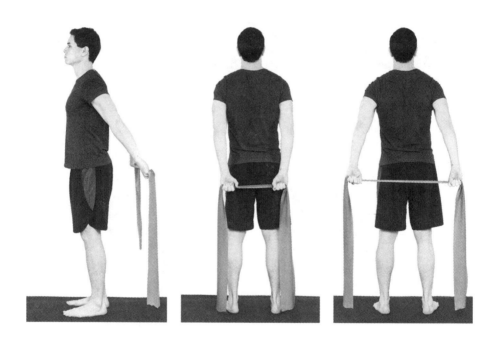

• • •

If you are at the gym, front latissimus pull-downs with a body bar in front, one-arm rows, pull-ups (assisted or not), and reverse flyes should be your choice exercises. Because you are suffering from core imbalance from too much forward hunch, you want to avoid benching or curling.

Please be smart when doing resistance training. Always keep abdominal muscles engaged when performing exercises and avoid overtraining, which can lead to injuries. With resistance training, your muscles need at least two days to recover, so five days of resistance training a week would be the maximum.

— DRINK UP! —

A great after-workout drink is milk. It has just the right amount of proteins and carbohydrates to inhibit muscle protein damage and reduce inflammation.

FREQUENTLY ASKED QUESTIONS

How many reps should I be doing?
Because our goal is great-looking abs, we want to do 12–15 repetitions. The more reps, the more fat we burn and the leaner our body gets.

And how many sets of repetitions?
Approximately three sets of 12–15 per exercise.

How long should my strength-training exercise routine be?
Thirty minutes is enough to build your strength and see results.

How often should I do resistance training?
About three days a week or every other day.

13.

CORE AND AB EXERCISES

THIS PLAN WILL give you alternatives to the dangerous crunch workout. But first, a patient story and how this workout was developed.

ONE PATIENT'S STORY

THERE ARE VERY FEW TIMES in one's professional life when you meet someone or learn something that is truly transformational. I can tell you what Dr. Sinett has to say in this book is truly transformational.

My name is Alex Torres, and I have been a Pilates instructor for the past 10 years, as well as a professional dancer for 15. I have worked with hundreds of clients to help them get core balance and fit-looking bodies. One of my clients recommended that I consult with Dr. Sinett.

Dr. Sinett started my examination by evaluating tension in my muscles and found my entire right side was significantly tighter than my left. From my jaw to my buttock and hamstring, it was all the same. He then went on to show me that my right hip was rotated higher than my left.

He checked my range of motion in my neck and showed that I could only turn about halfway of what I should. He then did some muscle testing that showed great function on my entire left side but weakness on my entire right side, including my abdominals (and I am right handed).

He went on to have me take the Core Imbalance Test. I turned my head to the right to see how far I could see (not very! I was tight!) and then again with my arm above my head (much further).

Dr. Sinett explained that I was suffering from core imbalance. While the exam made it indisputable, none of this made any sense to me. I am the one who helps clients get core balance. Aligning the spine while helping people exercise is what I was trained to do—or at least that is what I thought. Was it just because I had been exercising a lot? Dr. Sinett responded with a resolute no.

Dr. Sinett went on to explain that he felt equally baffled, until he discovered why most people suffered from this—even health professionals. He showed me how to put extension into my back, and my flexibility in my neck dramatically improved. All of the strength on my right side returned, including to my abdominals.

I left his office quite confused and excited at the same time. What I experienced was almost unbelievable but fascinating.

Dr. Sinett's information seemed 180 degrees different than everything that I had learned. I went back to Dr. Sinett to get some more answers to my questions and learn more about his theories.

Armed with the knowledge that any exercise that puts your body into flexion is harmful and that extension exercises are necessary, I changed my exercise routines. Immediately, not only was I feeling better, but my clients were as well. His theories were proving to be correct across the board.

Dr. Sinett then told me that he was writing his next book, titled *Sit-Ups Are Stupid, and Crunches Are Crap,* to share his information with the world and to teach people to properly

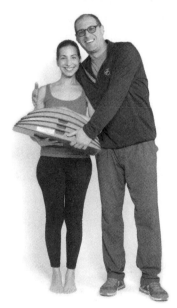

train their core and abs. I was excited that he asked for my help consulting on the core exercise section of the book. The workout we created for you is unparalleled in its simplicity and its ability to deliver great-looking abs—all while creating core balance.

—ALEX TORRES

■

THE AB AND CORE TRAINING PLAN

We must have proper balance between all of the core muscles, not just the ones that look good. The abdominal muscles and back muscles must work together to support our proper posture. These core-training exercises don't just work your abdominals but all of the supporting core musculature in a symmetrical and systematic fashion. A 2008 study in the *Journal of Strength and Conditioning* shows that exercises that extend your body while keeping your lower back in a safe, neutral position work the rectus abdominus 25 percent harder than crunches.

Training all of these muscles is much easier than you think and will ensure optimal results. The workout that follows will balance out your back muscles and engage your glutes, hamstrings, and quads, all while working your abdominals. Remember, proper training will also help prevent injuries rather than create them.

You can train your core up to five times a week. Always do your abdominal exercises at the end of your workouts because the abdominals are involved in almost any exercise. Having the abdominal muscles fatigued too early in your workout makes you much more susceptible to injury.

We recommend doing three different types of exercises for three sets per workout. Each set should contain approximately 10 to 12 repetitions.

Don't forget to exercise with proper form. This is much more important than the number of repetitions that you do (i.e., 7 reps with great form is better than 15 reps with increasingly poor form as you tire).

The exercises in this section range from beginner to advanced. Challenge yourself but be smart!

SEATED AND STANDING STRETCHES AND EXERCISES

THUMBS-TO-PITS STRETCH

■

You've heard of these first two stretches before, but we're including them again here because they are a great way to release your back as you are easing into a workout. Place your thumbs under your armpits with your fingertips pointed up to the ceiling. Now, tilt your head back and lift your thumbs up as high as possible. This stretch will open your chest and extend your mid-back.

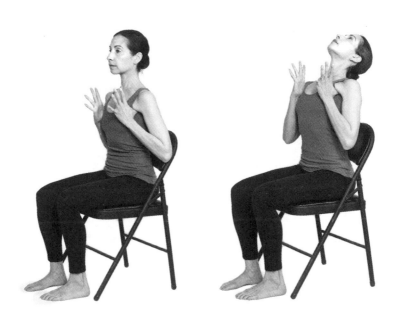

THE STANDING ABDOMINAL STRETCH

■

The standing abdominal stretch is a great way to make sure that you have the proper balance between flexion and extension. This stretch can be done anywhere and takes just seconds to do. Stand up, raise your arms above your head, and lean your torso backward.

We recommend doing them 15 times every hour. Do not go too far back—about a 30-degree angle will suffice. You should never feel pain while doing this. These stretches will relieve muscle soreness and tightness in your back, as well as dramatically improve your breathing.

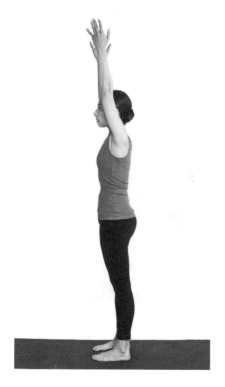
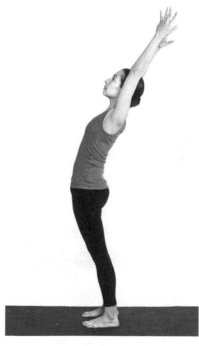

CALF STRETCH

■

Place your heels on the floor and your toes at the edge of the Backbridge or against a baseboard and lean in. Hold for 15 seconds and repeat three times.

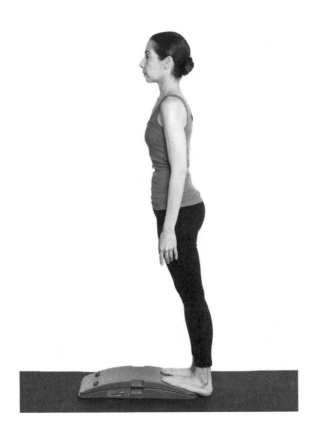

STANDING ABDOMINAL TWIST

■

Stand on your mat with legs wide, bend at your torso with your arms outstretched. Rotate your torso and let one arm raise straight up to the ceiling, while the other comes in contact with the floor. Switch sides and do 12 repetitions.

This is another good one for the obliques. If you are unable to reach the floor, you can use the Backbridge or a yoga block to raise your point of contact.

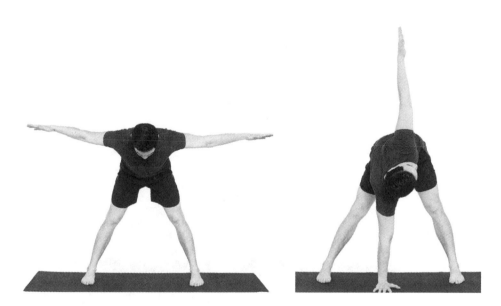

SQUAT

■

Stand with your feet at hips' width apart and slowly lower as if you are coming into chair pose. Rise back up to standing and repeat 12 times.

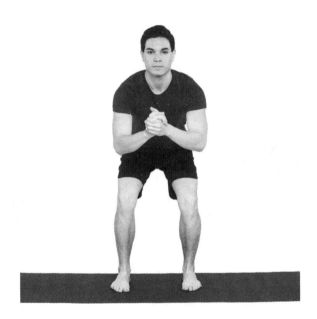

SUMO SQUATS

■

Spread your feet wider, and turn your toes out, so that they are in the eleven o'clock and one o'clock positions or even in the ten o'clock and two o'clock positions. Lower your hips down and then rise back up. Do 12 repetitions.

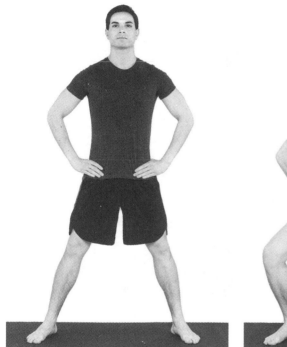
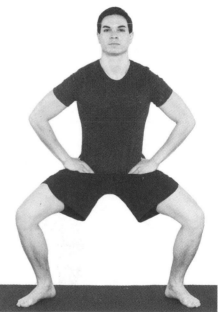

LUNGES

∎

Stand with your feet slightly separated and hands on your hips. Step one leg out in front and bend both knees as you sink into a nice lunge. Push off the front foot and come back to standing. Do 12 repetitions and then switch sides, so that the other leg steps out in front.

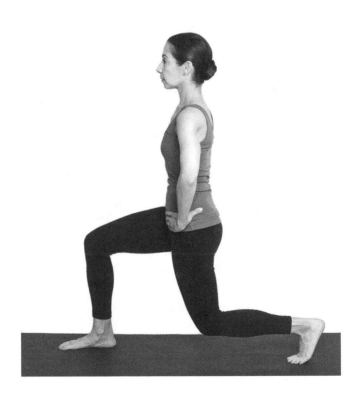

CORE EXERCISES
DONE ON YOUR BACK

SEATED TWISTS

■

Start by sitting on the floor, legs straight out in front of you. Bring both arms to one side of the floor next to you and then switch the arms to the alternate side.

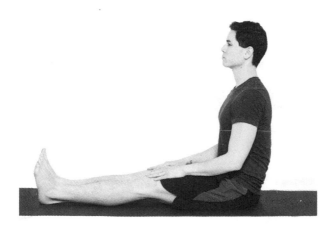

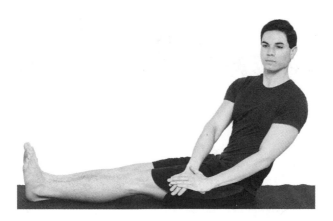

(continued)

To increase engagement of the abs, raise your legs and twist from side to side.

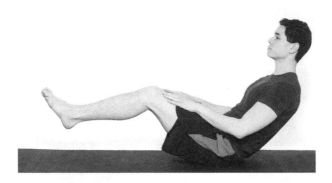

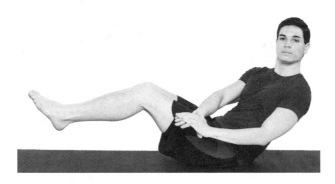

BOAT POSE

■

There are three variations of this pose, with increasing difficulty. Begin with Variation 1, sitting with knees bent and feet down. Grab the back of your knees and hold for a count of 10.

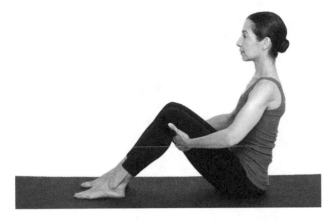

Variation 2 allows you to release the hands from the back of the knees and extend your hands out in front of you.

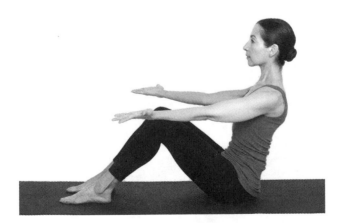

(continued)

For Variation 3, you'll lift your feet off the ground and hold the knees or keep hands extended.

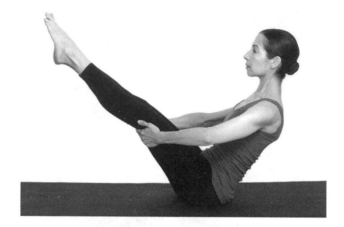

LOW BOAT POSE

■

Come into Variation 3 of Boat Pose, then lower your back so that just your shoulder blades are lifted and feet are slightly elevated from the floor. It's important that your back is straight and there is not too much "crunch." You can keep arms to your sides in line with your lifted legs or raise your arms overhead.

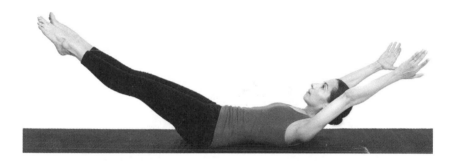

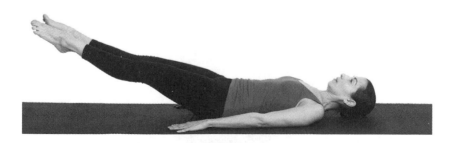

BRIDGES

∎

Lie flat on your mat with knees bent and feet on the ground. Slowly raise your hips and thrust your pelvis up toward the ceiling or sky. Hold for a count of 10 and then return to bridge position, adding in some leg variations. Extend one leg long in the air, hold the bridge, and then switch legs. You can also lift a bent knee in closer toward the chest and then lower it back to the ground.

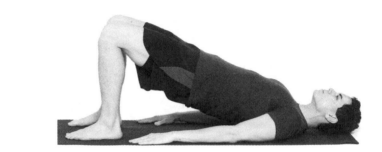

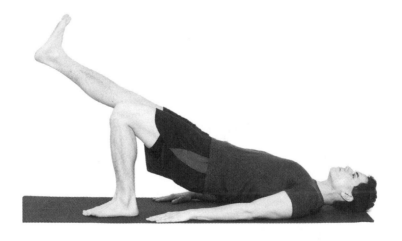

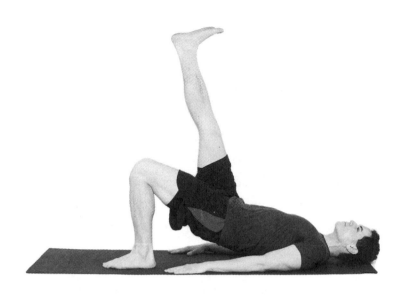

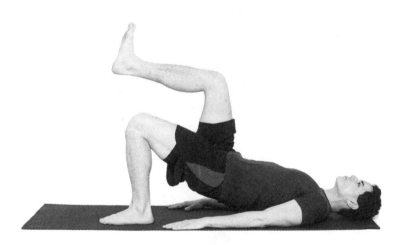

SKINNIES

■

A must for everyone! Skinnies work the transverse abdominus muscle. Lie on the floor, take a deep breath, and then let all of your air out and hold for a count of five while you draw your navel to the floor.

Repeat, go slow, and make sure that your breathing is steady. For a harder exercise, bend your knees and add some resistance by isometrically pushing your knees back with your hands. Never bring your neck up off the floor.

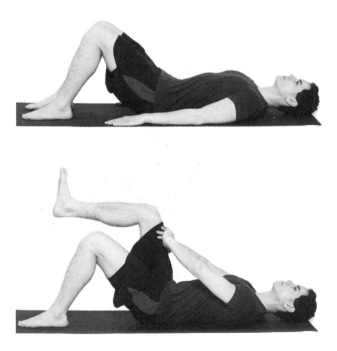

■

MARCHES

■

Stay in the same position as the skinnies and bring both knees to tabletop position. Lower one leg and then return it to table as you lower the other, so that it looks like you are marching in air.

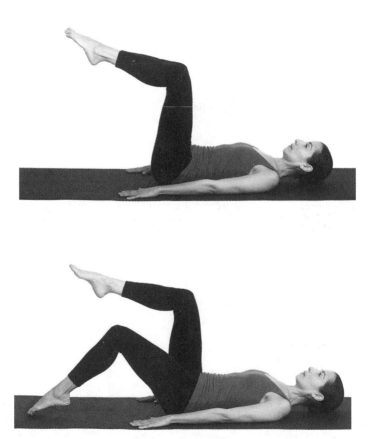

HALF BICYCLES

■

Lie on your back, bend your knees in the air, and then slowly extend them out one at a time and repeat. You can do them a little quicker, just as if you are riding a bike. Never bring your head and neck off of the mat.

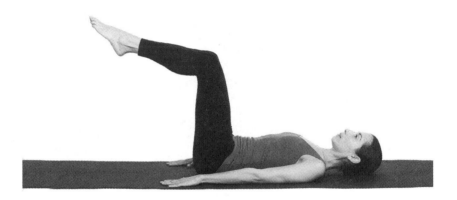

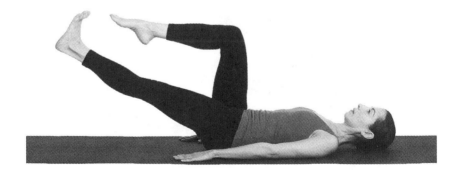

DEAD BUGS

∎

This exercise is similar to the Half Bicycles but adds arm movement. Start lying flat on the mat and bring your legs into tabletop position. Extend your arms straight in front of your chest. Extend your right arm over head and your left leg out long, then switch sides. Your legs will pedal like a bicycle, and your arms will be working, too.

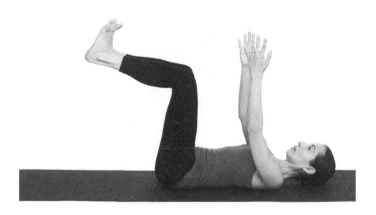

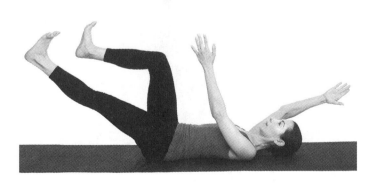

HIP-UPS

∎

Lie flat on your back. Gently lift your legs and hips to the ceiling, then hold for two seconds and repeat 12 times.

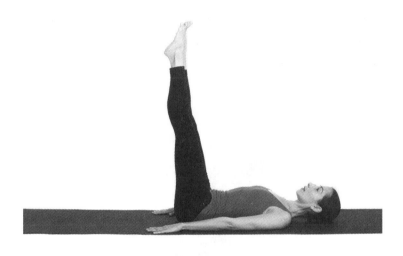

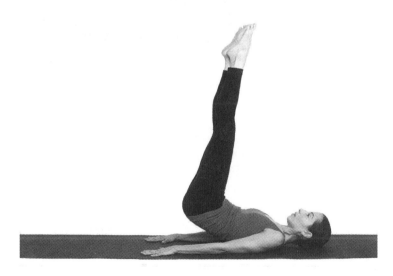

WINDSHIELD WIPERS–HALF AND FULL

∎

This exercise is a reclined twist with a boost and works your side or oblique muscles. Raise your legs with knees slightly bent and then slowly lower them to the side so that they touch the floor. If you are not able to reach the floor, go as far as you can go, then return to your starting point. Do 12 repetitions to one side (half wiper) and repeat on the other side.

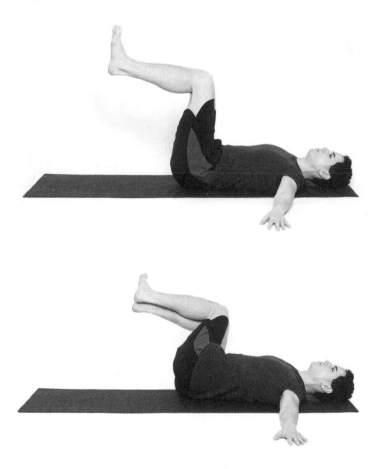

You can also try the full wiper, keeping your legs straight and twisting from side to side. Try to touch your feet to the ground or floor ever so slightly. Make sure that you have good form and control throughout the exercise.

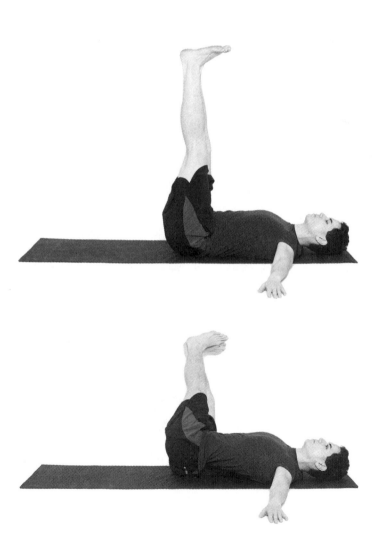

LEG RAISES

Lying on your back, raise both legs up about 70 degrees and then slowly lower them down. Repeat this 10 times.

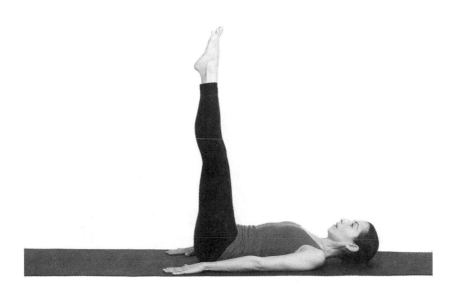

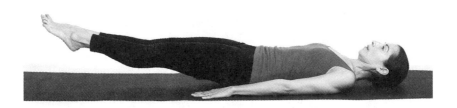

For a more isolated leg raise or to modify for your low back pain, place your buttocks on the Backbridge with your pelvis elevated, allowing for a greater range of motion. For a killer leg raise, try level 4 or 5. This will feel as if you are doing leg raises off the end of a bench, allowing a much greater range of motion and engagement of the abdominals.

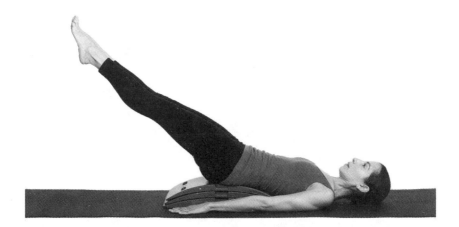

SPLITS, CIRCLES, AND SCISSORS

■

These are done the same way as the leg raise exercise, but you substitute raises for splits and small circles as you slowly go up and down throughout the range of motion—and add little flutter kicks for scissors.

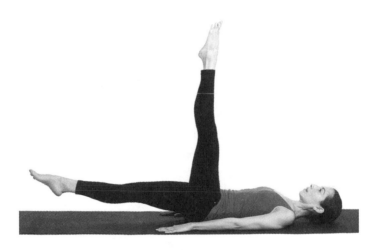

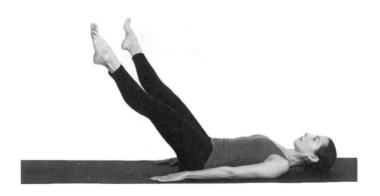

RECLINING TWIST

■

Keep your shoulders flat on the mat and pull both bent knees over your torso and place them on the floor. Hold the stretch for a minute and repeat on the opposite side.

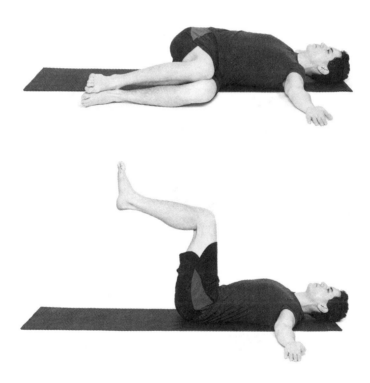

EXERCISES
LYING FACEDOWN

CAT COW

■

Lie on your belly on the mat and push up onto all fours in a table-top position. Gently round your back to come into Cat, hold for a count of five, and then slowly sink your belly and arch your back to come into Cow. Repeat until you feel ready to move on.

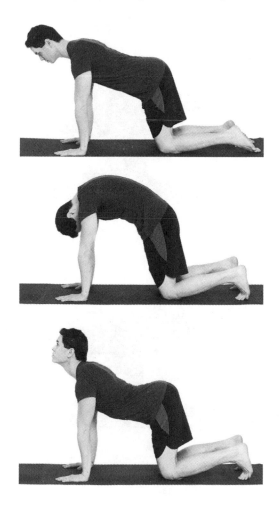

BIRD-DOG

■

Stay in tabletop position and lift your right arm off the floor and extend it. Then lift your left leg off the floor and extend it as well, so that you are balancing on your left hand and right leg. Switch sides.

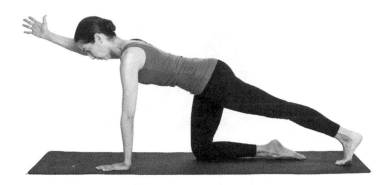

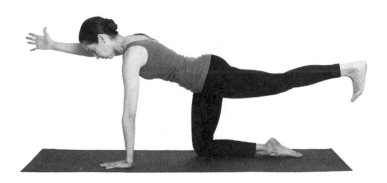

DONKEY KICKS

■

Still in tabletop position, lift one knee from the mat and kick it up, keeping the knee bent. Switch sides.

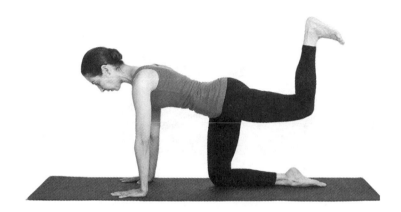

CHILD'S POSE

■

Sit on your knees and then lean forward, pulling your hips back. You can extend your arms out in front of you or keep your hands resting on the mat along your sides.

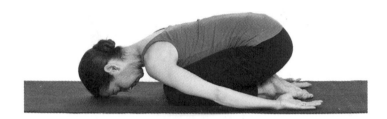

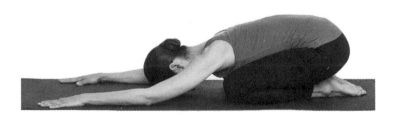

COBRA

■

Lying facedown, place your hands in front of you and do half a push-up, so that your upper torso is elevated but your pelvis still has contact with the floor. Raise your eyes to the ceiling or sky and hold for a count of five, then slowly lower yourself down and repeat.

This exercise works your lumbar extenders and lower back while stretching and lengthening the core. If doing the cobra with arms extended is too much for you, you can keep your forearms on the mat and just lift the chest for a smaller but still effective extension.

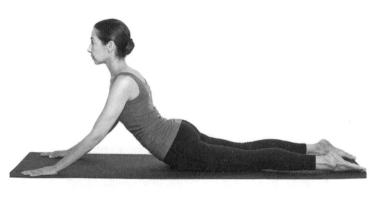

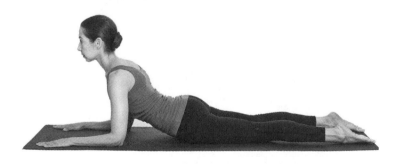

GOAL POST EXTENDERS

■

Lie on your belly and put your arms into goal-post form. Lift your torso off the matt and then slowly lower to starting position.

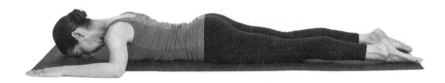

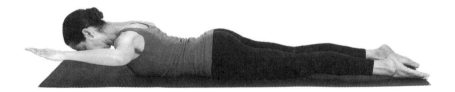

You can use the Backbridge if you want extra support.

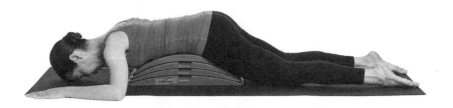

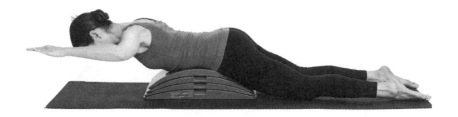

LUMBAR EXTENDERS WITH LOCUST HANDS

■

You will use the same form as the cobra exercise, but here you will interlock your hands behind your head. Extend back as far as you can, hold for a count of five, and release. Your feet will remain on the ground.

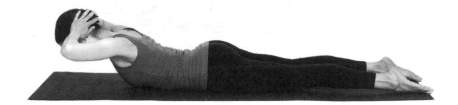

EXTENDERS WITH LOCUST ARM BIND

∎

Follow the previous exercise but join your hands behind your back and extend your arms. Then lower and rise for another count of five.

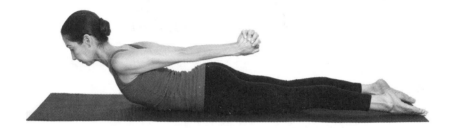

VS

■

Lying facedown, extend your arms like the letter V in front of you. Pull up to a cobra and hold for a count of five.

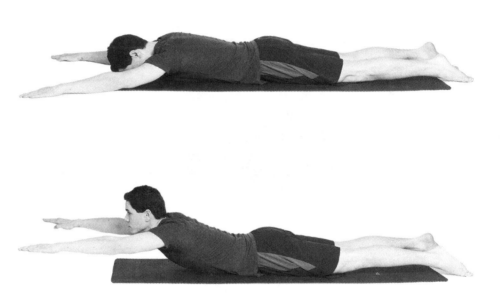

SUPERMANS

■

Still facedown, extend your arms and legs out. First try just elevating your arms, keeping your legs on the ground, and then try your legs with your arms down. After you have mastered this, elevate both your legs and arms at the same time and hold for counts of five.

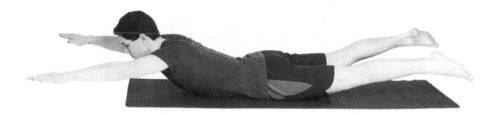

SWIMMERS

■

Stay in the Superman pose, but raise one arm and then switch.
Do the same by alternating legs. Then try fluttering your arms
and legs at the same time.

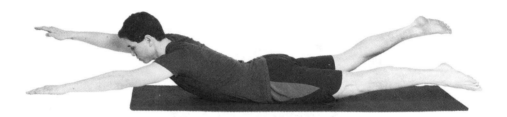

PLANKS

Plank is one of the best exercises for core work.

It keeps your spine aligned and doesn't introduce

any C-shape curve.

REGULAR PLANK

■

Lie on the mat on your belly with hands next to your shoulders. Tuck your toes under and push up, extending your arms. This is plank. Keep your neck aligned and your back straight. Do not drop your hips or round your spine. The goal is to slowly build up to one minute of holding plank.

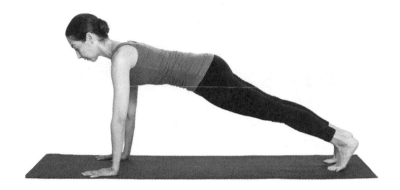

If this is too difficult to start, or if you need to alleviate pressure on your wrists, you can do a forearm variation. Lower your forearms to the floor and keep the rest of your body straight. You'll be in the same position, just lower on your arms.

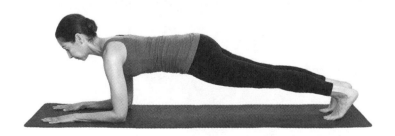

For an easier modification of plank, you can also keep your arms extended and drop your knees to touch the mat as you build strength and stability.

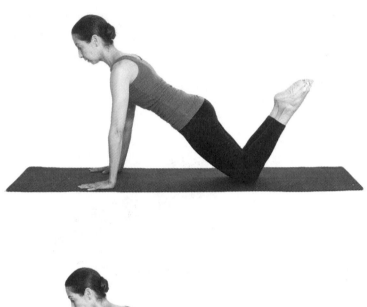

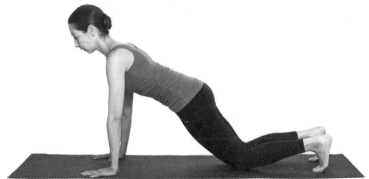

TWISTING PLANKS

■

This exercise works the oblique muscles. Hold the plank and then twist your pelvis, so that one side contacts the floor, while the other side is elevated. Return to center and turn the other way.

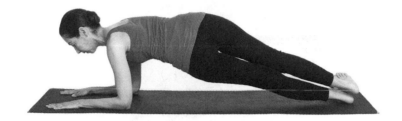

SHOULDER TAPS

■

Stay in plank position and lift one hand off the mat and bring it to touch the opposite shoulder. Return the hand to the floor and do the same by bringing the other hand to the other shoulder. Repeat 12 times. You can also add in the knees-down variation and do the shoulder taps from that position.

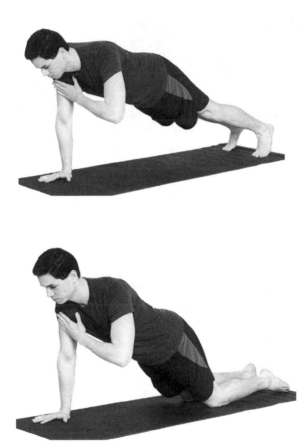

CROUCH

■

In plank position, lower your knees so that they are bent but lifted an inch or two off the floor. Hold for a count of 10.

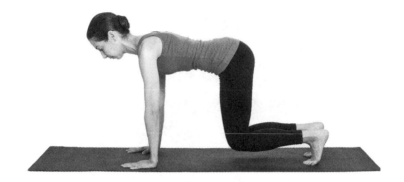

PUSH-UPS

■

Start in plank position and slowly lower to the ground, keeping elbows tucked into your sides. Push up and return to starting position.

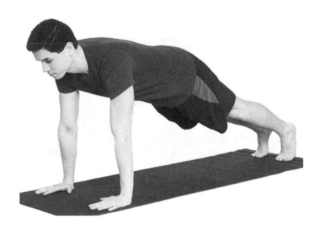

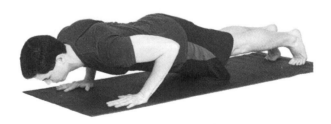

To modify, drop your knees to the ground and perform the push-up.

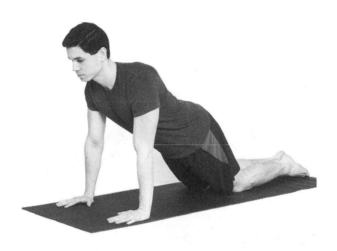

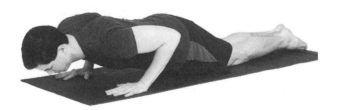

MOUNTAIN CLIMBERS

■

Start in a plank position. Bring one knee forward while holding the other in position and switch legs for 12 repetitions.

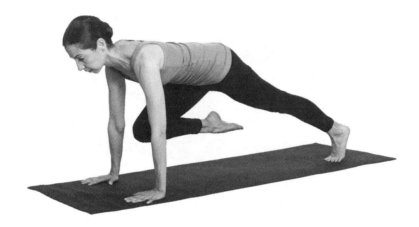

TWISTED MOUNTAIN CLIMBERS

■

Stay in regular mountain climber position. Bring one leg in and twist it across your body toward the opposite elbow. This works the obliques and gets your heart pumping.

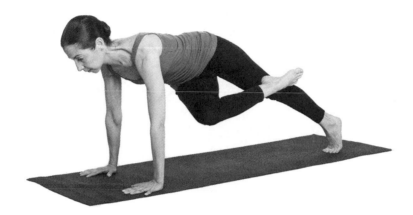

SIDE EXERCISES
AND STRETCHES

SIDE PLANKS

■

Lie on your side and place one forearm at 90 degrees while stacking your legs onto one another. Slowly elevate your hips so that your weight is on your forearm and the foot that is touching the ground. You can raise your top arm and extend it toward the ceiling or sky for stability.

If this is too much on your wrist, lower down to your forearm. Start by holding for a count of 10 and increase the hold as you progress. Then switch sides.

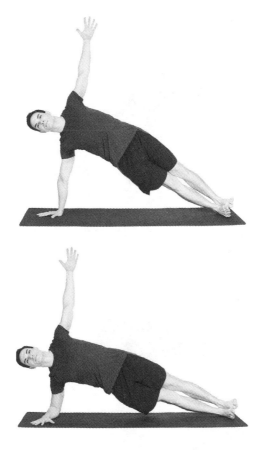

SIDE PLANK LEG VARIATIONS

■

Now try the side plank, with one arm either extended or the forearm on the ground, with leg variations. Stagger the feet. Then stagger the feet and lift the top leg to about 70 degrees. Do 12 reps, raising and lowering the leg, while holding the side plank. Try dropping the bottom knee to support you if it gets to be too intense.

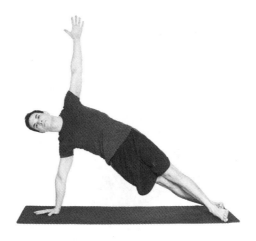

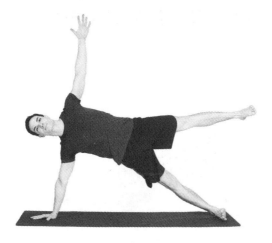

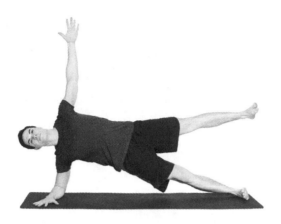

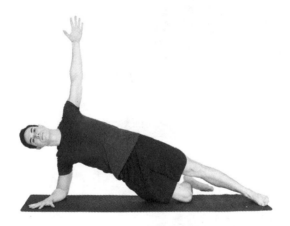

THREAD THE NEEDLE

■

In side plank position, with lower arm extended or forearm on the mat, raise your upper arm up to the ceiling or sky and then pass your top arm under the opposite arm. You'll get a bit of a twisting motion in the core as you "thread the needle."

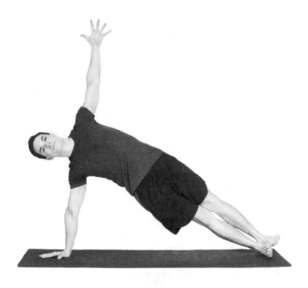

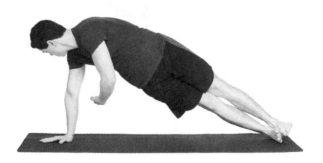

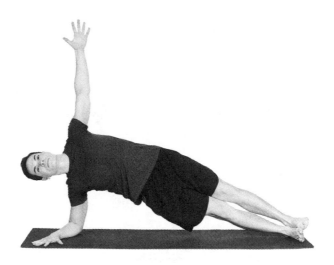

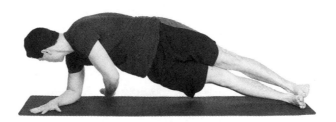

DIAMONDS

Lie on your side propped up on your bottom forearm. Raise your top leg, keeping knee bent, so that the space between your legs forms a diamond shape.

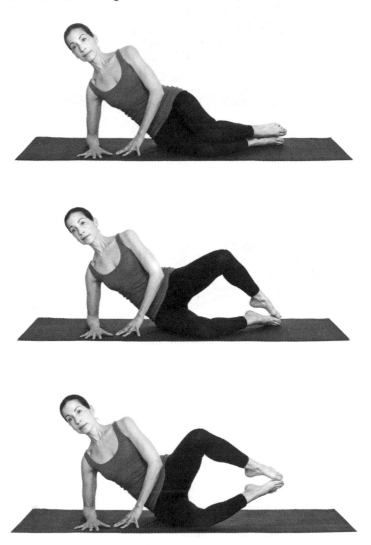

For a variation, lie on your side with your bottom arm extended beneath you. Hold and switch sides.

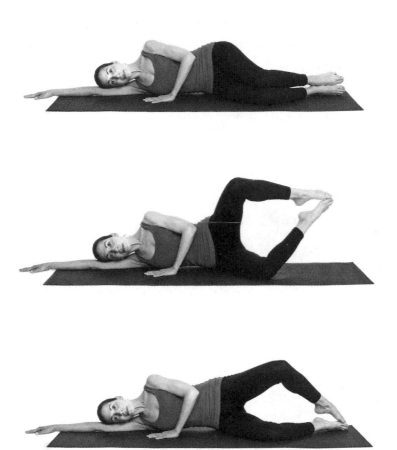

LEG RAISES

■

Lie on the mat on one side. You can prop your head up with your bottom hand, or you can extend your lower arm down to the ground and rest your head on your arm. Slowly raise the top stacked leg, keeping the bottom leg stable on the floor. Do 12 repetitions and switch sides.

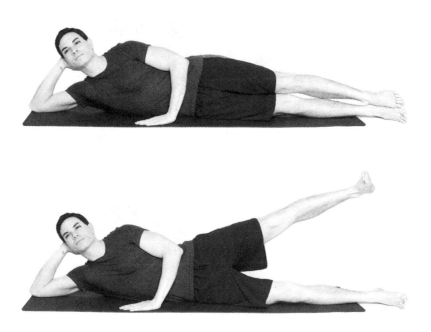

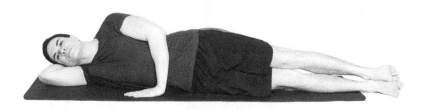

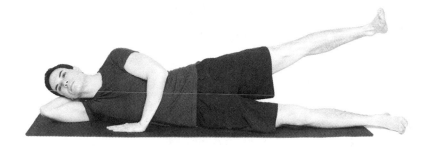

CHEST OPENER

■

You learned how to do the Backbridge version of this on page 79, but you can also do this one by lying on your side on a mat. It's a great way to open up after all these side exercises. Bring your knees into your chest, so that they make a 90-degree angle. Extend your arms out straight in front of you and then lift and open the top arm, lowering it to the floor on the opposite side as you shift your gaze toward the outer arm.

14.

HEALTHY EATING
THE FLAT ABS EATING PROGRAM

DIET AND FAT-BURNING exercises together are key. One without the other is not nearly as effective. You could have the strongest abdominals in the world, but no one will see them unless you have a lean waist.

While I'm not behind fad diets, I am fully behind healthy eating—and a *big* part of seeing those ab muscles emerge is how you eat. Whether you're looking to show off in a swimsuit, reduce your risk for dangerous diseases, or just feel better, my eating plan is for you. Here is how to tackle the fourth prong of six-pack abs: healthy eating.

■

DON'T DIET

The first three letters in the word diet spell *die*, as in "This diet is killing me!" Dieting is a multibillion-dollar industry and one that completely boggles my mind. I certainly understand the need for people to look their best, and from the ever-increasing rates of cosmetic surgery, I see that people are willing to pay large sums of money and go through immense pain all to look better. However, the sad statistical facts in the case of diets is that they do not work.

Nearly 65 percent of dieters regain lost weight within three years, according to Gary Foster, Ph.D., clinical director of the Weight and Eating Disorders Program at the University of Pennsylvania.* And statistics also say that only 5 percent of crash dieters keep the weight off.

With dieting, people are pursuing the wrong solution. What is important to realize in weight loss is that your weight is not your problem. Yes, you read that right. Weight is not your problem!

Your additional weight is the result of your unhealthy habits, not the cause of it. If you are trying to lose weight, you are chasing the tail and not the source. The source is the bad and habitual choices you make on a daily basis—your unhealthy lifestyle, if you will.

My eating plan and principles help you correct the root of the problem and teach you how you can reveal your ab muscles using a premier approach that tackles the hard-to-target belly region on three levels: zapping excess fat, decreasing bloating, and reducing water retention. So, not only are you melting away belly fat, you're also minimizing circumstances that could create bloating and puffiness and make your middle look bigger. It

---

* https://www.livestrong.com/article/438395-the-percentage-of-people-who-regain-weight-after-rapid-weight-loss-risks/.

will not involve starvation or deprivation. You will eat delicious meals . . . and snacks . . . and dessert.

So, let's blast some belly fat!

THE BASICS:
THREE PRINCIPLES FOR
EATING FOR FLAT ABS

PRINCIPLE ONE: TRIM THE EXCESS FAT

No matter how fab your ab muscles are, they'll never get the attention they deserve if they're covered up with excess fat. You've got to minimize belly fat to let those ab muscles shine. There are three incredibly powerful ways to zap belly fat:

1. Cut the Refined Foods

Which would be a more satisfying snack, a deli-sized bag of pretzels or a slice of whole grain toast with 1 tbsp hummus, $\frac{1}{4}$ of a sliced avocado, three slices of tomato, plus a handful of baby carrots? The toast snack is a larger volume of food, has more flavor, and a combination of textures. Would you believe that the toast with hummus and veggies actually has *fewer calories* than the pretzels? It would take you at least twice as long to enjoy it, provides more nutrition (including satiating protein, iron, and calcium), and is a whole lot more flavorful.

You can't lose weight without reducing your calorie intake, but that doesn't mean eating "diet" foods and depriving yourself.

Cutting out refined white flour foods and foods with gobs of added sugar means more room in your diet for foods that fill you up on fewer calories, like beans, whole grains, fruits and veggies, and low-fat dairy. You'll feel like you're eating more, but you'll be shedding extra fat at the same time.

2. Kick It Up a Notch

Those spicy red peppers that add serious heat to your food do more than just make you reach for a cold beverage. Turns out that the pungent compound found in those spicy peppers, called capsaicin, is pleasantly surprising researchers on a regular basis. Studies printed in *Chemical Senses* in 2012 and *Appetite* in 2014 have found that spicing up your meals with hot pepper can increase your body's calorie-burning capacity, suppress your desire for fatty, sweet, and salty foods, and reduce mindless eating. Wow!

With results like that, it shouldn't surprise you that I spiced up my flat abs diet. You'll see ways to add spice to the meals and snacks on my plan, denoted with a "kick it up" label. If you're not into flaming-hot flavors, start slow—sprinkle just a dash of cayenne onto a sandwich or add just a touch of spicy pepper to your tomato sauce.

Or, if you like things spicy, then by all means turn up the heat. The bottom line is that eating your spicier meals might mean a smaller bottom line on you . . . and more quickly emerging ab muscles.

3. Make Room for MUFAs

What is a MUFA, you ask? It's a monounsaturated fat, meaning that the chemical structure of the fat has a double bond in one of its chains of fatty acids. For our purposes, MUFAs are healthy fats that reduce cholesterol and are linked to decreasing belly fat.

That's right, eating fat is linked to a reduction in belly fat. For those of you who are still living in the fat-free zone, it's time to start embracing fats in your diet again. Not only are MUFAs specifically related to less abdominal fat, but you need fat in your diet to help your body absorb certain vitamins, like vitamins A, D, E, and K.

Plus, fat gives your meals and snacks a more satisfying feel and delivers delicious flavor. Remember, you eat more when something doesn't satiate you. A small amount of healthy fat will actually save you calories in the long run. You'll certainly find healthy MUFAs in my meal plans thanks to delicious, nutritious foods like nuts, seeds, avocados, olives and olive oil, canola oil, and whole grains.

PRINCIPLE TWO: BEAT THE BLOAT

If you're walking around feeling puffy, full, and bloated, chances are you're not going to be super confident about showing off your abs, not to mention the fact that you're probably feeling uncomfortable a lot of the time. That's no fun for anyone. But if you experience bloating frequently, you're not alone.

Belly bloating is most often a result of water retention or gas, a buildup of air in the intestines and/or the stomach. In order to minimize it, there are some key things you must do;

1. Stop Overeating

It might sound obvious, but bloating is not caused by one food or one group of foods in particular but rather by chronically overeating at each meal. Many of my patients find that their symptoms disappear once they cut back to smaller, more frequent meals with more appropriate portion sizes.

Have you ever skipped a meal, only to become ravenously hungry and then overeat when you do finally have a meal? This scenario is all too common.

The first step to fixing this is mapping out more structured meals and snacks, and eating at designated times. I recommend that my patients start by aiming to eat five to six times per day. A great way to make sure this happens is by writing down your eating plan for a week, including all meals and snacks, in addition to a general idea of what it might be. Follow your plan for a couple days, seeing what works and what doesn't for your appetite, stomach, and exercise-fueling needs, then adjust as you need to for the next week. After doing this for a few weeks, you'll not only likely see a difference in your bloating but also in your energy level and your weight.

Another popular trick for eating less is eating off a smaller plate. The theory is that your portion looks bigger on a smaller plate, and this tricks your mind into thinking you are eating more food. Eating and hunger is often emotional, and this simple switch can sometimes help reset your perception of what a serving size really is.

USE THE HUNGER SCALE

Another very helpful tool to naturally eating appropriate portion sizes is something called the hunger scale. The hunger scale is a scale from 1 to 10 that offers a way to rate your hunger: 1 is ravenously hungry, and 10 is so stuffed you're feeling drowsy and an urgent need to slip into some looser pants.

When to start eating: At a 3 on the scale, you should be feeling the beginning signs of hunger, just before your stomach actually starts rumbling. This is where you want to start a meal or snack. In other words, you never want to let yourself get so hungry that you're feeling ravenous, light-headed, or have a growling stomach. If you have these hunger symptoms, you've gone too far and have a greater chance of overeating at your next meal or snack.

When to stop eating: If you want to lose weight, stop eating at a 5. This is a neutral point where you don't feel hungry anymore, and though you could still eat more without being stuffed, you feel satisfied. If you are looking to maintain your weight, you can stop eating at a 6–7, which is where you'd be just past the satisfied point of feeling not hungry. You're full enough to

(continued)

---

keep from falling back down to a 3 for the next two to three hours but can also comfortably move around without loosening your pants.

One of the things that the hunger scale helps with is being more mindful when you're eating in general. So even throughout the course of your meal, take a pause to evaluate how your hunger levels rank.

Another good test to make sure that you aren't overeating is the treadmill test, which means that, at any point in the day, you should be able to go on a treadmill to exercise. If you need to rest and digest after a meal, it means you overate.

2. Slow Down

Let's face it. We're all guilty of eating a meal or two too fast while working, getting the kids ready, etc. But eating too quickly, especially while multitasking, can add stress and extra gulps of air to your meal—both of which can lead to bloating.

Slowing down at meals can help, even if it's just setting aside 10–15 minutes to sit down, focus on eating, and be more mindful of your body. A study at the University of Rhode Island in 2011 found that when 30 female subjects ate the exact same meal twice, they consumed 70 fewer calories when they made an effort to eat more slowly and chew their food thoroughly than when they ate at their usual pace.

3. Eat Enough Fiber, But Not Too Much

While getting enough fiber is super important for keeping your digestive system healthy and regular, getting too much can also make bloating worse. Women should aim for approximately 25–30 grams of fiber per day and men a range of 30–38 grams.

And when it comes to fiber, strive to get it the natural way, from whole foods like fruits, veggies, whole grains, and beans, rather than packaged foods that have added fiber. For instance, granola bars that are not 100 percent whole grain but that have fiber added just to make them higher in fiber should be passed up for the 100 percent whole grain variety.

In order to spot added fiber, look for ingredients like inulin and chicory root listed. If a product that isn't whole grain boasts lots of fiber, you can be pretty sure it's coming from added fiber and is best avoided. When you do eat foods that are high in fiber, make sure that you're drinking plenty of water to help promote smoother digestion and prevent any fiber-related bloating.

4. Manage Stress

Your emotions play a large role in your metabolism. Sound surprising? Just think about it: this theory explains why some people can consume very few calories and not lose weight, while others can eat significantly more and never gain a pound.

Our bodies produce chemicals when we're under stress. One such chemical is cortisol, and high levels of it can lead to that hard-to-get-rid-of belly fat. So, if you eat a hot fudge sundae to celebrate an achievement, your body has a completely different biochemical response than if you were to eat the sundae while you are depressed (or if you then beat yourself up about eating a hot fudge sundae).

This is exactly why many diets don't work. Depriving people of food joys can lead to unhappiness and resentment—two very unhealthy emotions, which can increase your cortisol levels and affect the way you process the foods you do eat.

When it's related to a condition called Irritable Bowel Syndrome (IBS), bloating can also often be worsened by chronic stress. It's important for everyone—with IBS or not—to manage the stress in their lives for a multitude of health reasons, both mental and physical. Whether it is planning a weekly yoga and/or meditation session, making time to relax with your family, or writing down your weekly goals, stress management should be a part of your flat abs plan.

5. Nix Sugar Alcohols

Despite the name, sugar alcohols are neither sugar nor alcohol. They are, in fact, a type of carbohydrate that sweetens foods, but they have fewer calories (about half) than sugar, and they can cause serious bloating in people who are sensitive to them.

There are many different types of sugar alcohols that are used in foods, most of them ending in "-ol," such as maltitol, erythritol, sorbitol, and xylitol. Sugar alcohols are most often found in foods that are marketed as "low in sugar" or "sugar free." So, if you're consuming many foods with this label (especially sugar-free gum, sugar-free ice cream, or other sweets like pancake syrup), you are likely consuming sugar alcohols on a regular basis. The best way to find out is to check out the ingredients labels.

6. Avoid Carbonation

Whether it be a soda or a sparkling water, anything that has carbonation can create gas and bloating. If you want a beverage, choose water.

PRINCIPLE THREE: REDUCE WATER RETENTION

1. Spare Some Sodium

Excess sodium makes your body retain water, leaving you feeling puffy. Dining out or regularly eating packaged convenience foods makes for a diet that's too high in sodium. The typical American consumes an average of 3,400 mg of sodium per day, compared to the recommended 2,300 mg per day by the US Dietary Guidelines of 2010.

One of the first things you can do to minimize the amount of sodium in your diet is to start eating out less and making more of your meals from whole foods rather than packaged. Basing meals and snacks on fruits, vegetables, lean proteins (like chicken, fish, and beans), whole grains, and low-fat dairy also helps to lower blood pressure.

When you do buy staple packaged foods, choose lower sodium options in foods like salsa, tomato sauce, bread and bread products, breakfast cereal, cheese, lunch meat, and frozen meals. You can use the following as general guidelines:

Salsa: no more than 150 mg sodium per two tbsps

Tomato sauce: no more than 350 mg per ½ cup

Bread: no more than 160 mg per slice

Breakfast cereal: no more than 250 mg per serving

Cheese: no more than 200 mg per slice

Lunch meat: no more than 360 mg per two ounces

Frozen entree: no more than 700 mg

2. Pack in Potassium

While sodium causes water retention, potassium is a natural counter to this, helping to prevent water retention. Fortunately, including more high potassium foods in your diet isn't too difficult. Potassium is found in many fruits and veggies, some protein sources, and beans.

At the top of the list are winter squash, sweet potatoes, white potatoes, white beans, nonfat/low-fat yogurt and milk, bananas, cantaloupe, and salmon. The recommended Daily Value for potassium is 3,500 mg per day, and the foods listed here contain at least 10–20 percent of the Daily Value of potassium per serving.

3. Include Protein with Every Meal

Making sure that you have protein with each meal and snack can work wonders for water retention. Protein acts as a natural diuretic to help your body get rid of extra fluid. Avoid carb-heavy meals and instead include protein, healthy fats, and some whole grains in each meal.

For instance, for breakfast, you might have an egg sandwich on whole grain toast with avocado and salsa. The flat abs meal plans included in the next chapter all meet protein requirements for each meal and snack.

4. Stay Hydrated

Being properly hydrated makes every organ in your body work more efficiently. And when it comes to banishing puffiness, drinking water will help flush waste out of your system—and that includes extra water.

As a general rule, you can aim for approximately eight cups (64 ounces) of water each day. However, when the weather is very warm or you are exercising for long periods of time, you may need more than this.

The best indicator for hydration is to measure the color of your urine. If it's clear to lemonade-like, you're likely adequately hydrated. If it looks like apple juice or darker, get drinking.

In order to remind yourself to keep hydrated, it's wise to invest in a BPA-free water bottle that you can carry everywhere with you. In addition, fruits and veggies are actually packed with water, too, especially watermelon, which is why it's also one of the flat abs super foods.

10 SUPERFOODS FOR SLIM ABS

The following foods contain key components that I have outlined in this chapter. Some are excellent sources of MUFAs, fiber, potassium, and hydration, while others help you eat a larger volume of food for fewer calories in order to blast fat from your abs. These foods are incorporated into the flat abs meal plans that follow.

Blueberries: With just 84 calories and a whopping four grams of fiber per cup, blueberries are also rich in antioxidants that help improve blood flow. This means more oxygen is delivered to muscles during your workouts, maximizing the fat-blasting effect that you get from them.

Watermelon: As its name implies, watermelons are packed with water, making them very hydrating. Being well hydrated is important for the functioning of every system in your body, including your metabolism. Watermelon is also super low in calories, with just 46 calories per cup—lower than most other fruits—so it makes a great ab-friendly sweet treat.

Avocado: Avocado is considered a fat in your meal plans, so it's ironic that it actually helps your body blast belly fat.

But research shows that monounsaturated fats, which avocados contain lots of (roughly 10 grams per avocado), help fight ab fat when incorporated as part of a healthful diet.

Lentils: These little legumes are rich in iron, another nutrient that is important for carrying oxygen to your muscles during cardio and ab workouts. On top of that, lentils have a combination of a hefty dose of fiber (8 grams per $\frac{1}{2}$ cup) and protein (8 grams per $\frac{1}{2}$ cup), which makes them ideal for keeping your blood sugar more balanced and preventing an imbalance of hormones that can lead to higher ab fat.

Quinoa: This tiny grain (that's actually a seed) is a source of complete protein and contains all of the amino acids our bodies need to repair and build muscle. It's also loaded with B vitamins, which help your body convert the food you eat into energy.

Natural nut butters (peanut, almond): Peanut and almond butter are rich in monounsaturated fats (MUFAs), just like avocados. Nut butters also pack in a lot of flavor and a creamy texture, both of which can make a simple meal or snack feel more satisfying.

Salmon: This cold-water fish is one of the best sources of Omega 3 fatty acids, which are not only linked to improved heart health and decreased inflammation but also might help your body burn more fat (rather than store it). Getting adequate Omega 3s has also been linked to improved cognition.

Spicy foods: Capsaicin (the natural chemical in hot peppers that gives them their heat) can give you a small metabolism boost. One study indicated the capsaicin in red pepper might help you feel more satisfied and eat less. Plus, we tend to eat spicier foods slower, which can also help you eat less.

Air-popped popcorn: Three cups of air-popped popcorn contains under 100 calories and more than three grams of fiber, making this a smart, satisfying snack for anyone trying to shed extra weight or just snack smarter. The fiber helps you feel fuller, and the sheer volume of the snack promotes satisfaction.

Refrigerated Sauerkraut: Sauerkraut is a fermented food that provides probiotic bacteria, fiber and powerful antioxidants. Just make sure it's refrigerated, meaning it hasn't been canned with heat to create shelf stability, so all that good bacteria is still active!

15.

FLAT AB MEAL PLANS

THESE MEALS ARE equally tasty and healthy, helping to maximize your fat-burning potential while minimizing bloating and water retention. Mix and match any breakfast with any lunch, dinner, snack, and treat to make up your daily plan.

There are seven of each, which means there are lots of combinations that you can make. Some of the meals also contain a "kick it up" suggestion, which is a way to add a little calorie-burning spice to many of the meals.

• • •

BREAKFASTS
(300 CALORIES)
■

APPLE PECAN CEREAL

1¼ cups spoon-size shredded wheat

½ cup 1 percent milk (or dairy alternative)

½ chopped apple

1 tbsp chopped pecans

dash of cinnamon

Top cereal with milk, apple, pecans, and cinnamon, and enjoy!

ANTIOXIDANTS ON-THE-GO

½ cup very strong green tea

1 cup 1 percent milk (or dairy alternative)

1 tsp maple syrup

dash of powdered ginger

Heat tea and mix with milk, syrup, and ginger. Eat with ¼ cup unsalted almonds mixed with 1 tbsp dried cherries.

This meal may not sound like much, but so many people skip breakfast altogether, and a grab-n-go light meal or snack like this will help tide you over and give you satiating protein, so that you don't overeat or resort to fast food as you head to work.

AVOCADO BREAKFAST TOAST

1 slice whole grain bread

2 tbsp hummus

¼ sliced avocado

1 hardboiled egg

Toast bread and top with hummus, avocado, and sliced egg. Sprinkle with black pepper and salt.

Kick it up: Sprinkle with cayenne pepper.

BLUEBERRY-WALNUT CEREAL

¾ cup cooked quinoa

½ cup blueberries

⅓ cup 1 percent milk (or milk alternative)

1 tbsp chopped walnuts

1 tsp honey

¼ tsp cinnamon

Combine ingredients and enjoy!

FLAT AB BREAKFAST SMOOTHIE

1 cup 1 percent milk (or dairy alternative)

1 cup raw spinach

¼ cup chopped carrot

½ banana, ½ cup frozen or fresh blueberries

¼ avocado

dash of cinnamon

Combine ingredients in a blender. Add ice to desired consistency.

EGG AND VEGGIE SCRAMBLE

1 tbsp chopped onion

¼ cup chopped bell pepper

¼ cup grape tomatoes

1 tsp olive oil

1 egg and 2 egg whites

salt, pepper, and cumin (a pinch of each)

½ cup rinsed and drained black beans

1 tbsp chopped avocado

Sautee onion, pepper, and tomatoes in olive oil for about four minutes. Whisk eggs and add to the pan with salt, pepper, cumin, and black beans. Cook until firm, about another four minutes. Top with avocado and enjoy!

Kick it up: Add a pinch of cayenne when you add the cumin, salt, and pepper.

ALMOND BUTTER AND APPLE

Another quickie but goodie. Spread each half of an apple with 2 tsp almond butter and 2 tbsp granola. Sprinkle with a dash of pumpkin pie spice.

LUNCHES
(450 CALORIES)
■

SESAME VEGGIE SLAW WITH CHICKEN AND BROWN RICE

1 cup thinly sliced purple cabbage

¼ cup diced carrot

2 tbsp chopped red onion

1 tbsp hemp seeds

1 tbsp store-bought sesame dressing

1 cup diced grilled skinless chicken breast

½ cup cooked brown rice

Toss purple cabbage with carrot, red onions, hemp seeds, and the dressing. Pour over grilled chicken and brown rice.

Kick it up: Add a pinch of fresh, diced chili to the dressing.

5-MINUTE CORN AND BEAN CHILI

1½ cups reduced sodium tomato soup

1 cup corn

¾ cup rinsed and drained kidney beans

a pinch of chili powder

1 tbsp chopped avocado

pinch of fresh cilantro

Combine ingredients and heat in the microwave or over medium heat in a saucepan until steaming. Top with avocado and fresh cilantro.

Kick it up: Stir a dash of hot pepper sauce into the soup while it's heating.

CURRIED EGG SALAD ON CRACKERS

2 hard-boiled eggs and 2 hard-boiled egg whites

2 tbsp chopped celery

2 tbsp chopped carrot

1 tbsp chopped green onion

1 tbsp chopped cashews

1 tbsp golden raisins

2 tsp reduced fat mayonnaise

2 tsp nonfat plain Greek yogurt

⅛ tsp curry powder

pinch of salt and pepper

2 whole grain crisp bread crackers

Chop hard-boiled eggs and whites, and mix with the celery, carrot, green onion, cashews, and golden raisins. Whisk together mayonnaise and nonfat plain Greek yogurt with curry powder and salt and pepper. Stir the dressing into the egg mixture. Serve with bread crackers.

Kick it up: Add a pinch of cayenne to the mayonnaise mixture.

TEMPEH TOSS

½ cup crumbled tempeh

1 tsp olive oil

1 cup broccoli slaw

¾ cup cooked quinoa

1 tbsp balsamic vinegar mixed with ½ tsp Dijon mustard

1 tbsp sunflower seeds

1 tbsp chopped dried apricots

Sautee tempeh in olive oil until hot. Toss with the broccoli slaw, cooked quinoa, balsamic vinegar, Dijon mustard, sunflower seeds, and dried apricots.

Kick it up: Instead of Dijon mustard, mix a dash of hot sauce and a pinch of salt into the vinegar.

WHOLE GRAIN SALAD WITH SALMON

1½ ounces canned wild salmon, drained

1 cup cooked barley or brown rice

½ cup halved grape tomatoes

½ cup chopped cucumber

1 tsp capers

2 tsp red wine vinegar

½ tsp dried oregano

2 tsp olive oil

Toss wild salmon with barley or brown rice, grape tomatoes, chopped cucumber, capers, red wine vinegar, dried oregano, and olive oil.

Kick it up: Add a pinch of cayenne to the mixture before tossing all ingredients together.

GRILLED PORTOBELLO BURGER WITH ROASTED PEPPER

1 Portobello mushroom cap
1 tsp olive oil
whole grain hamburger bun
2 tbsp hummus
¼ cup sliced roasted red pepper
1 slice of Swiss cheese

Brush the Portobello mushroom cap with olive oil and broil or grill until tender. Spread hummus on top half of the bun. Layer mushroom, red pepper, and Swiss cheese on bottom half of the bun.

Kick it up: Stir a dash of hot sauce into the hummus before spreading on bun.

CINNAMON, PEANUT BUTTER, AND APPLE WRAP

2 tbsp peanut butter
10-inch whole grain tortilla
dash of cinnamon
dash of ground ginger
1 apple

Spread the peanut butter on the tortilla and sprinkle it with the cinnamon and ginger. Thinly slice half of the apple, place on top of the peanut butter, and roll up. Serve with the other half of the apple.

DINNERS
(450 CALORIES)
■

CHILI-TOPPED SWEET POTATO

1 large sweet potato

1 cup reduced-sodium vegetarian chili

¼ cup chopped tomato

1 tbsp nonfat plain Greek yogurt

1 tbsp chopped avocado

Bake sweet potato until tender all the way through for about 45 minutes in a 400-degree oven. Then, top with the vegetarian chili, tomato, Greek yogurt, and avocado.

Kick it up: Stir a pinch of cayenne into the chili before adding to the potato.

FLANK STEAK RICE BOWL OVER ARUGULA

3 ounces thinly sliced flank steak

2 tsp olive oil

4 tsp lime juice

1 tsp chopped garlic

¼ tsp chili powder

¾ cup brown rice

¾ cup cooked corn kernels

a pinch of garlic powder

2 tsp freshly chopped cilantro

2 cups arugula

Toss the steak with 1 tsp olive oil, 2 tsp of the lime juice, garlic, and chili powder. Sautee steak over medium-high heat until cooked to your liking. Toss the brown rice with the corn kernels, the rest of the lime juice, 1 tsp olive oil, garlic powder, and cilantro. Make a bed of arugula on a plate and top with corn mixture and beef.

Kick it up: Drizzle hot sauce over the top of the salad after you layer the steak on.

CHICKEN, BULGUR, AND BROCCOLI BOWL WITH LEMON VINAIGRETTE

¾ cup skinless chicken breast

1 cup cooked bulgur wheat

1 cup roasted broccoli

1 tbsp freshly chopped parsley

2 tsp olive oil

2 tsp lemon juice

dash of salt and pepper

Grill the chicken breast, then toss with the bulgur wheat, broccoli, parsley, olive oil, and lemon juice. Season with salt and pepper to taste.

Kick it up: Mix a pinch of cayenne in with the other ingredients.

ROASTED POTATO WITH GREENS AND A POACHED EGG

1 large Russet potato

4 tsp olive oil

pinch of salt and pepper

2 cups mixed greens

2 tsp balsamic vinegar

½ tsp chopped garlic

1 poached egg

Chop the potato and toss with 2 tsp of the olive oil and a pinch of salt and pepper. Roast at 400 degrees for about 20 minutes until soft. Toss 2 cups mixed greens with the remaining 2 tsp olive oil, 2 tsp balsamic vinegar, and ½ tsp chopped garlic. Place the roasted potato on top of the dressed greens and top with 1 poached egg.

Kick it up: Add hot sauce to the oil mixture and toss potatoes before roasting.

COLLARDS AND PORK TENDERLOIN PASTA TOSS

½ cup sliced bell pepper

2 cups roughly chopped collard greens

¼ cup diced onion

1 tbsp olive oil

4 ounces grilled or baked pork tenderloin

1 cup cooked whole wheat rotini

2 tsp chopped toasted walnuts

Sautee the bell pepper, collard greens, and onion in 1 tbsp olive oil until soft. Grill or bake 4 ounces of pork tenderloin, then cut into strips and toss meat and vegetables with the pasta. Sprinkle toasted walnuts.

Kick it up: Add a pinch of cayenne to the veggies when sautéing.

TUNA PITA PIZZA

6-inch whole wheat pita

2 tsp olive oil

⅓ cup marinara sauce

5-ounce can (drained) tuna

⅓ cup frozen and thawed artichoke hearts

¼ cup part-skim mozzarella cheese

Brush the pita with the olive oil and top with marinara sauce, tuna, artichoke hearts, and mozzarella cheese. Place in a 400-degree oven for about 10 minutes until cheese is melted and golden.

Kick it up: Sprinkle the marinara with a pinch of cayenne before adding other toppings.

ROASTED EGGPLANT AND BEAN BURRITO

10-inch whole wheat tortilla

1 cup pinto beans, rinsed and drained

1 tbsp salsa

½ cup roasted eggplant

¼ cup chopped avocado

Top the tortilla with all the ingredients, roll up, and bake at 350 degrees for about 10 minutes until heated through.

Kick it up: Drizzle a dash of hot sauce over the avocado before rolling up.

SNACKS
(150 CALORIES)

■

- Top 6 ounces nonfat plain Greek yogurt with ½ cup sliced grapes and a tsp chopped crystallized ginger.

- Veggie chips: 1 ounce Terra chips and a glass of water with lemon and cucumber slices.

- Trail mix and tea: 3 tbsp trail mix and a cup of green tea.

- Freeze-dried fruit pack: 1 ounce package of Funky Monkey Bananamon freeze-dried snacks and 7 almonds.

- Tropical watermelon: 1½ cups cubed watermelon topped with 1 tbsp dried coconut.

- Salt-and-pepper popcorn: 3 cups popcorn tossed with 1 tsp olive oil and a pinch of salt and pepper. *Kick it up*: Add a dash of hot sauce.

- Avocado with a kick: Half an avocado drizzled with 1 tsp lemon juice and a dash of chili powder. *Kick it up*: Use cayenne instead of chili powder.

TREATS
(150 CALORIES)
■

It's important to include treats—foods that you love but that don't contribute any considerable nutrition value—in any diet plan. Cookies, brownies, sweetened drinks, candy, refined carbohydrate foods like white bread or crackers, and alcohol are all considered treats. Giving yourself a treat every day helps you from feeling deprived. Remember, you are not dieting, just learning how to eat healthfully. A treat is healthy for the mind and soul, and a proper portion won't throw your body off.

This meal program includes about 150 calories per day from treat foods. The foods listed below are examples that you can follow. Feel free to substitute 150 calories of any other treat food in place of these:

Hot chocolate: 6 ounces hot 1 percent milk (or dairy alternative) with 2 Hershey's Kisses stirred in until melted

Dark chocolate fix: 3 squares of 60-percent-or-higher dark chocolate

Night out: 6 ounces of wine or a 12-ounce light beer

Sweet treat: a 2-inch square brownie

To-go: half a Justin's Organic Dark Chocolate Peanut Butter Cup

Donut shop: 2 doughnut holes

Out to eat: 1 small dinner roll with 1 tsp butter

Learning how to eat, what to eat, when to eat, and how much to eat is vital to getting the abs you always dreamed of. A special thanks to Willow Jarosh and Stephanie Clark from C and J Nutrition, who created these wonderful meals and the nutritional advice for this section.

THAT'S A WRAP!

WE HAVE BEEN getting the wrong information from our fitness trainers and doctors, and we deserve the truth about health and fitness. Of course, we need strong abdominal muscles to support our back, but the sit-ups and crunches previously prescribed have no stabilizing factor for the back and are causing more harm than good. Large amounts of flexion exercises lead to postural imbalances that have a harmful and far-reaching negative effect on our overall health. Muscles need to contract and relax, not just continually contract.

We should no longer be swayed by marketers to purchase abdominal equipment that is based on a false premise of "spot reducing" and great-looking models. Overweight people should no longer attempt to lose their guts by doing sit-ups and crunches. Athletes should no longer train improperly and suffer non-contact injuries.

Rather, we should all approach our bodies and our health in a sensible manner by taking the four-pronged comprehensive approach I have detailed. No one can achieve the results that they are looking for without incorporating aerobic exercise, resistance training, core-stabilizing abdominal exercises, *and* a healthy diet. The exercises and meal plans that I have included for you are the best way to get and maintain lean abs and a balanced core. They will help you function optimally without risking injuries and alleviate a lot of your aches and pains.

After reading this book, I hope you'll never do a sit-up or crunch again.

Remember, the rect..s abdominus (the six-pack) is *not* the only important abdominal muscle and getting rid of crunches does *not* mean getting rid of the promise of flat abs. Flat abs are important, and not just because they look good.

Don't forget these important points for core health as you move forward with your new ab-conscious lifestyle:

- Most adults need a 35-inch-or-less waist for a male and a 34-inch-or-less waist for a female to have a healthy core.
- Consistency is key. Create your own exercise routine that works for you and your time schedule.
- Spot training does not work. You must focus on the whole package.
- Do the Backbridge every day to remove your daily flexion brought on by hours of sitting. If you don't have a Backbridge, use a yoga ball or try the standing

abdominal stretch and thumbs-to-pits stretch to add extension to your spine.

- The solution to pain created by your current workout is extension exercises. The solution to your pain from your sedentary lifestyle is extension exercises.

For more videos, information, and workouts, visit my websites at drsinett.com and backbridge.com. And don't forget to keep taking the Core Imbalance Test as you progress in your workouts to be sure that you are maintaining balance and proper form, and preventing those nasty non-contact injuries as you move forward in life and fitness.

Here's to your core and more!

Dr. Todd Sinett

INDEX

INDEX

INDEX

INDEX